T0110123

Allergies

Fight Them
with
the Blood
Type Diet®

Also by Dr. Peter J. D'Adamo with Catherine Whitney

Eat Right 4 Your Type: The Individualized Diet Solution to Staying Healthy, Living Longer, and Achieving Your Ideal Weight

Cook Right 4 Your Type: The Practical Kitchen Companion to Eat Right 4 Your Type

Live Right 4 Your Type: The Individualized Prescription for Maximizing Health, Metabolism, and Vitality in Every Stage of Your Life

Eat Right 4 Your Baby: The Individualized Guide to Fertility and Maximum Health During Pregnancy, Nursing, and Your Baby's First Year

Eat Right 4 Your Type Complete Blood Type Encyclopedia

Blood Type O: Food, Beverage and Supplement Lists

Blood Type A: Food, Beverage and Supplement Lists

Blood Type B: Food, Beverage and Supplement Lists

Blood Type AB: Food, Beverage and Supplement Lists

Dr. Peter J. D'Adamo Eat Right 4 (for) Your Type Health Library

Arthritis: Fight It with the Blood Type Diet®

Cancer: Fight It with the Blood Type Diet®

Cardiovascular Disease: Fight It with the Blood Type Diet®

Diabetes: Fight It with the Blood Type Diet®

Fatigue: Fight It with the Blood Type Diet®

DR. PETER J. D'ADAMO

WITH CATHERINE WHITNEY

Dr. Peter J. D'Adamo's

Eat Right 4 Your Type

Health Library

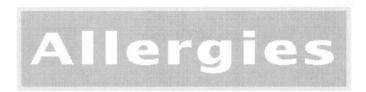

Allergies

Fight Them
with
the Blood
Type Diet®

BERKLEY BOOKS

NEW YORK

THE BERKLEY PUBLISHING GROUP
Published by the Penguin Group
Penguin Group (USA) Inc.
375 Hudson Street, New York, New York 10014, USA
Penguin Group (Canada), 90 Eglinton Avenue East, Suite 700, Toronto, Ontario M4P 2Y3, Canada
(a division of Pearson Penguin Canada Inc.)
Penguin Books Ltd., 80 Strand, London WC2R 0RL, England
Penguin Group Ireland, 25 St. Stephen's Green, Dublin 2, Ireland (a division of Penguin Books Ltd.)
Penguin Group (Australia), 250 Camberwell Road, Camberwell, Victoria 3124, Australia
(a division of Pearson Australia Group Pty. Ltd.)
Penguin Books India Pvt. Ltd., 11 Community Centre, Panchsheel Park, New Delhi—110 017, India
Penguin Group (NZ), cnr Airborne and Rosedale Roads, Albany, Auckland 1310, New Zealand
(a division of Pearson New Zealand Ltd.)
Penguin Books (South Africa) (Pty.) Ltd., 24 Sturdee Avenue, Rosebank, Johannesburg 2196,
South Africa

Penguin Books Ltd., Registered Offices: 80 Strand, London WC2R 0RL, England

PRINTING HISTORY
G. P. Putnam's Sons hardcover edition / April 2005
Berkley trade paperback edition / January 2006
Berkley trade paperback ISBN: 978-0-425-20753-6

The Library of Congress has cataloged the G. P. Putnam's Sons hardcover edition as follows:

D'Adamo, Peter.
    Allergies : fight them with the blood type diet / Peter J. D'Adamo with Catherine Whitney.
        p.   cm.—(Eat right 4 your type health library)
    Includes index.
    ISBN 0-399-15252-0
    1. Allergy—Alternative treatment.   2. Blood groups.   I. Whitney, Catherine (Catherine A.).
II. Title.
RC588.A47D33   2005   2004060038
616.97'06—dc22

DEDICATED TO THOSE
WHO ARE OPEN TO FINDING
NEW WAYS TO TREAT OLD ILLS

Acknowledgments

THIS BOOK OFFERS THE BEST THAT NATUROPATHIC MEDICINE and blood type science have to offer in the prevention and treatment of allergies. It has been a collaborative process, and I want to express my deep thanks to the people who have been involved in its creation.

I am most grateful to Martha Mosko D'Adamo, not only my partner in life and in parenting but also my partner in bringing the valuable wisdom about blood type to the world. Martha daily provides love, support, insight, and inspiration to all of my endeavors.

Catherine Whitney, my writer, and her partner, Paul Krafin, are invaluable word masters who have once again captured exactly the right tone in tackling this complex topic.

My literary agent and friend, Janis Vallely, always takes time to listen and advise. Her quiet guidance and personal support make the work possible.

I would also like to acknowledge others who have made significant contributions to my work: my colleague Bronner Handwerger, N.D., whose research and clinical abilities are deeply appreciated; Heidi Merritt, who continues to make an important contribution to the work; John Harris, whose knowledge and input have been invaluable; Laura Mittman, N.D., FIFHI, who has been such a big help in my efforts to educate other professionals; and Catherine's agent, Jane Dystel, who provides consistent support.

Amy Hertz, my former editor at Riverhead/Putnam, was the force behind the blood type books. My new editor, Denise Silvestro, continues to guide the work with dedication and skill.

As always, I am extremely grateful to the wonderful staff at Riverhead Books and Putnam. They have been tireless and enthusiastic, and their efforts have made it possible to continue bringing this important work to the market.

PETER J. D'ADAMO, N.D.

Contents

Allergies

Fight Them
with
the Blood
Type Diet®

New Tools
to Fight
Allergies

THE BLOOD TYPE DIET CAN BENEFIT EVERYONE. YOU don't have to be sick to see the effects. But most of the people who come to my clinic or contact my Web site are dealing with a serious chronic disease, or have received a distressing medical diagnosis. They want to know how they can hone the general guidelines of the Blood Type Diet to target their illness. Dr. Peter J. D'Adamo's *Eat Right 4 Your Type Health Library* has been introduced with these people in mind.

Allergies: Fight Them with the Blood Type Diet allows you to take full advantage of the medicinal benefits of eating and living according to your blood type. If you think of the standard Blood Type Diet as the foundation, the guidelines in this book provide a more targeted overlay for people who want to act aggressively to treat allergies. These dietary and lifestyle adaptations, individualized by blood type, supply additional ammunition to your allergy-fighting arsenal. They attack the problem at its source, restoring balance to your immune system, reducing inflammatory activity, and making you more keenly aware of specific environmental and dietary factors that trigger allergic reactions.

Here's what you'll find that's new:

- A disease-fighting category of blood type–specific food values, the **Super Beneficials,** emphasizing foods that have medicinal properties for treating allergy-related conditions.
- A more detailed breakdown of the **Neutral** category to limit foods that are known to have less nutritional value or may cause allergic reactions. Foods designated **Neutral: Allowed Infrequently** should be minimized or avoided.
- Detailed supplement protocols for each blood type that have been calibrated to support you at every stage of your battle with allergies. They include **Immune System Health Maintenance, Anti-Inflammatory/Allergy Relief, Sinus Relief, Digestive System Repair,** and **Adrenal Support.**
- A **4-Week Plan** for getting started that emphasizes what you can do right now to improve your condition and start feeling better right away.
- Plus many strategies for success, quizzes, checklists, and the answers to the questions most frequently asked about allergies at my clinic.

The chemistry of blood type continues to provide important clues to the biological and genetic mechanisms that control health and disease. In more than twenty-five years of research and clinical practice, I have successfully treated thousands of patients suffering from environmentally triggered or food allergies. Increasingly, medical doctors and naturopaths throughout the world are applying the blood type principles in their practices, with remarkable results.

I urge you to talk to your physician about the benefits of incorporating individualized, blood type–specific diet, exercise, and lifestyle strategies into your current plan. I am confident that employing the guidelines in this book will place you on the road to recovery. Take the step now, and use your blood type to your best advantage.

Why Blood
Type Matters

YOU ARE A BIOLOGICAL INDIVIDUAL.

Have you ever wondered why some people are constitutionally frail and susceptible to infection, while others seem naturally hardy? Why some people are able to lose weight on a particular diet, while others fail? Why some people age rapidly and show early signs of deterioration, while others are full of vitality into their later years?

We are all different. A single drop of your blood contains a biochemical signature as unique to you as your fingerprint. Many of the biochemical differences that make you an individual can be explained by your blood type.

Your blood type influences every facet of your physiology on a cellular level. It has everything to do with how you digest food, your ability to respond to stress, your mental state, the efficiency of your metabolic processes, and the strength of your immune system.

You can greatly improve your health, vitality, and emotional balance by knowing your blood type and by incorporating blood type–specific diet and lifestyle strategies into your health plan.

Be the biological individual you were meant to be!

What's Your Blood Type– Allergy Risk?

General Risk Factors (all blood types)

The following factors are known to contribute to allergies in sensitized individuals. Answer yes or no to each question, then total the values of the "yes" answers.

Risk Factor	Yes	Value
Has one or both of your parents had allergies?	☐	2
Does your job involve the use of chemicals (e.g., photocopying toners) or latex products (e.g., rubber gloves)?	☐	2
Do you live and/or work in a poorly ventilated building?	☐	1
Are you exposed to pesticides on your property or in your neighborhood?	☐	2

Is there a high mold count in your area? (This information is available from the National Allergy Bureau; see Appendix C for contact information.)	☐	1
Do you smoke, or live/work with smokers?	☐	3
Does your diet regularly include highly processed and frozen foods?	☐	2
Do you have a history of antibiotic use?	☐	3
Are you obese (more than 30% overweight)?	☐	2
Do you have an autoimmune disease?	☐	3

Total the number of "yes" answer points (21 points maximum)

The Blood Type O Quiz

The following factors are known to specifically influence Blood Type O's susceptibility to allergies. Answer yes or no to each question, then total the values of all "yes" answers.

Risk Factor	Yes	Value
Are you a non-secretor? (See page 27.)	☐	3
Do you generally follow a high-carbohydrate, low-protein diet?	☐	3
Do you regularly consume wheat or corn products?	☐	3
Do you regularly consume dairy products?	☐	2
Do you eat a lot of nightshade vegetables (tomatoes, potatoes, eggplant, etc.)?	☐	1
Do you have any gastrointestinal problems, such as ulcers, ulcerative colitis, or irritable bowel syndrome?	☐	2
Do you suffer from inflammatory problems, such as rheumatoid arthritis?	☐	3
Is your level of aerobic exercise under four hours weekly?	☐	3

Total the number of "yes" answer points (20 points maximum)

Scoring: Total the values of "yes" answer points in both quizzes.

25–41: High to Very High Risk. You already have or are very likely to develop allergies. Take immediate action with adherence to the Blood Type Diet and modify the factors that are in your control.

12–24: Moderate to High Risk. If you make some diet and lifestyle changes, you may alleviate the symptoms of allergies, or avoid them altogether. Refer to your blood type section to determine which actions you must take.

1–11: Low to Moderate Risk. Your overall susceptibility to allergies is relatively low. Keep it that way by adhering to the Blood Type Diet and lifestyle plan.

The Blood Type A Quiz

The following factors are known to specifically influence Blood Type A's susceptibility to allergies. Answer yes or no to each question, then total the values of all "yes" answers.

Risk Factor	Yes	Value
Are you a non-secretor? (See page 27.)	☐	3
Do you regularly follow a high-protein, high-fat diet?	☐	3
Do you eat wheat once or twice a day?	☐	2
Do you eat dairy foods every day?	☐	1
Do have a high stress job or family environment?	☐	2
Do you avoid exercise, even stretching or yoga?	☐	3
Do you easily succumb to infections, colds, and flu?	☐	2
Do you suffer from digestive problems, such as gastrointestinal reflux or celiac disease?	☐	3

Total the number of "yes" answer points (19 points maximum)

Scoring: Total the values of "yes" answer points in both quizzes.

25–40: High to Very High Risk. You already have or are very likely to develop allergies. Take immediate action with adherence to the Blood Type Diet and modify the factors that are in your control.

12–24: Moderate to High Risk. If you make some diet and lifestyle changes, you may alleviate the symptoms of allergies or avoid them altogether. Refer to your blood type section to determine which actions you must take.

1–11: Low to Moderate Risk. Your overall susceptibility to allergies is relatively low. Keep it that way by adhering to the Blood Type Diet and lifestyle plan.

The Blood Type B Quiz

The following factors are known to specifically influence Blood Type B's susceptibility to allergies. Answer yes or no to each question, then total the values of all "yes" answers.

Risk Factor	Yes	Value
Are you a non-secretor? (See page 27.)	☐	3
Do you regularly follow a high-carbohydrate, low-fat diet?	☐	3
Do you regularly consume wheat or corn products?	☐	2
Do you regularly consume any of the following foods: chicken, buckwheat, peanuts, lentils?	☐	3
Do you suffer from anxiety or depression?	☐	1
Do you have a history of urinary or reproductive tract infections?	☐	2
Do you have a history of viral infections?	☐	3
Is your total weekly exercise time under four hours?	☐	3

Total the number of "yes" answer points (20 points maximum)

Scoring: Total the values of "yes" answer points in both quizzes.

25–41: High to Very High Risk. You already have or are very likely to develop allergies. Take immediate action with adherence to the Blood Type Diet and modify the factors that are in your control.

12–24: Moderate to High Risk. If you make some diet and lifestyle changes, you may alleviate the symptoms of allergies or avoid them altogether. Refer to your blood type section to determine which actions you must take.

1–11: Low to Moderate Risk. Your overall susceptibility to allergies is relatively low. Keep it that way by adhering to the Blood Type Diet and lifestyle plan.

The Blood Type AB Quiz

The following factors are known to specifically influence Blood Type AB's susceptibility to allergies. Answer yes or no to each question, then total the values of all "yes" answers.

Risk Factor	Yes	Value
Are you a non-secretor? (See page 27.)	☐	3
Do you regularly follow a high-protein, high-fat diet, with little or no soy or cultured dairy?	☐	3
Do you regularly consume chicken or corn?	☐	3
Do you eat wheat once or twice a day?	☐	2
Is your total weekly exercise time under four hours?	☐	3
Do you easily succumb to infections, colds, and flu?	☐	2
Do you suffer from gastrointestinal problems, such as gastrointestinal reflux or celiac disease?	☐	3

Total the number of "yes" answer points (19 points maximum)

Scoring: Total the values of "yes" answer points in both quizzes.

25–40: High to Very High Risk. You already have or are very likely to develop allergies. Take immediate action with adherence to the Blood Type Diet and modify the factors that are in your control.

12–24: Moderate to High Risk. If you make some diet and lifestyle changes, you may alleviate the symptoms of allergies or eliminate them altogether. Refer to your blood type section to determine which actions you must take.

1–11: Low to Moderate Risk. Your overall susceptibility to allergies is relatively low. Keep it that way by adhering to the Blood Type Diet and lifestyle plan.

PART I

Blood Type and Allergies: A Basic Primer

The Dynamics of Allergies

THE WORD *ALLERGY* MEANS "ALTERED WORKING." IT WAS coined at the beginning of the twentieth century, after dogs inoculated with proteins from other animals had severe reactions when they came into contact with those proteins again.

Allergies are responses mounted by the immune system to a particular food, inhalant, or chemical. In a simplified sense, an allergic reaction is an adverse or inappropriately amplified immune system response to something that many other people find harmless. Most commonly, an allergic reaction expresses itself as a headache or fatigue, and may include sneezing, watery eyes, and nasal congestion. More severe allergic reactions, such as those to certain nuts, fish, and insect stings are known as anaphylaxis and are characterized by the swelling of tissue and the inability to breathe. These reactions may need to be treated as serious medical emergencies. A synthetic epinephrine, a hormone naturally produced by the adrenal gland, may be administered to combat the reaction. People with severe allergies should carry epi-nephrine pens in case of accidental exposure to the allergen.

Systemic Effects of Allergies

RESPIRATORY	asthma
	bronchitis
	hay fever (allergic rhinitis)
	sinusitis
SKIN	eczema (atopic dermatitis)
	hives
	rash
	acne
DIGESTIVE	celiac disease
	colitis
	Crohn's disease
	irritable bowel syndrome
	leaky gut syndrome
	bladder infection
OTHER	ADHD
	ear infection
	chronic fatigue syndrome
	anaphylactic shock

According to the National Institute of Allergy and Infectious Diseases (NIAID), people with allergies spend more than $5 billion annually on doctors' visits, allergy shots, and prescription medications. Many health conditions are related to allergies, including acne, asthma, attention deficit disorders, bladder infections, and a host of digestive disorders.

System Overload

WHY ARE SOME PEOPLE allergic and others not? While allergies are quite complex physiologically, to simplify it, the difference between a person suffering from allergies and one who is free and clear is a matter of the total load on the system. This is particularly true of seasonal allergies. In a sense, we are all like camels. We can carry a certain burden without our backs giving way and collapsing. The burdens we carry are the shared burdens of all creatures, like environmental pollution and toxins. Individually, we may carry the burdens of poor diet, stressful relationships or jobs, lack of sleep, over- or underexercise, and any number of medical conditions. If your total load is reaching its maximum capacity, and then an additional bundle—such as seasonal pollen exposure—is tossed on your back, you will collapse. It literally becomes the straw that breaks the camel's back. So allergy avoidance is often a matter of reducing the total load. That's one reason why the Blood Type Diet is so effective against allergies. It removes a great deal of the burden you carry, allowing you to support the added weight of environmental burdens more easily.

Diet's crucial role goes well beyond resolving specific food allergies. More than half of your immunologic activity is located in your digestive system. When you consume the proper diet for your blood type, you build systemic immunity.

Inside an Allergy Attack

YOUR IMMUNE SYSTEM can be likened to a modern army, composed of many different divisions that operate under the direction of a central command. Like the military, the immune system requires good intelligence. It must identify and attack the enemy, while at the same time preventing casualties from "friendly fire."

In a properly functioning immune system, B- and T-lymphocyte cells are responsible for detecting invaders and producing antibodies against them. When B-cells encounter something they perceive as foreign to the body—such as a bacteria, virus, etc.—they become plasma cells and secrete large quantities of antibodies. The antibodies are specific to the antigen and neutralize the foreign agent or destroy it. T-helper cells are involved in this response. TH-1 helper cells enhance the ability of the immune system to respond to infections or injury.

TH-2 helper cells increase antibody production by releasing growth factors that increase antibody production. When these T-helper cells become overactive, they produce the immune system equivalent of friendly fire. No longer able to distinguish between friend or foe, they destroy the cells of "self."

The allergic reaction is related to this hyperactive response. The immune system of an allergic person reacts defensively when a particular allergen is present, producing large quantities of a special class of antibodies called immunoglobulin E (IgE). Different IgE antibodies are produced for each type of allergen, whether it's latex, pet dander, oak pollen, or ragweed pollen. IgE molecules are specific for the original allergen and can readily bind to the allergen that caused their production.

These allergen-specific IgE molecules travel through the blood and attach to receptors on the surface of mast cells—cells found in most body tissues, which synthesize and release histamine, a chemical that produces the classic symptoms of watery eyes, sneezing, welts, and hives. Once allergen-specific IgE has attached to the mast cell surface, it can remain for weeks or even months, always ready to bind to the original allergen. The next time the original allergen enters the body, the allergic cascade begins, and again results in the release of histamines from the mast cell. The symptoms may occur in just minutes, or up to an hour after contact.

People seem to inherit allergies, most often from their mothers. At least three genes are believed to be responsible for allergies, but only one has been identified. This gene produces interleukin 4 (IL-4), a growth factor that is required for production of IgE. Overproduction of IL-4 leads to more production of IgE, which in turn leads to an allergy.

Most attacks are defensive reactions of the immune system against certain innocuous substances that the body mistakes for harmful parasites. IgE is found to increase greatly in response to a parasitic infection. Eosinophils (cells that kill parasites such as worms) work in conjunction with IgE. Thus, one of the classic signs of a child with parasites is an itchy nose and watery eyes—a result of the immune system trying to kill a parasite and meanwhile liberating enough IgE to mimic the symptoms of allergy.

Non-Caucasians tend to have higher levels of IgE than others, and males tend to have higher levels than females. Levels of IgE tend to drop with aging, which may explain why some people grow out of childhood allergies.

As a rule, people with inherited skin diseases, including eczema, have a genetic predisposition for developing IgE antibody-mediated hypersensitivity to inhaled and ingested substances. These allergens are harmless to people who do not have the predisposition. This isn't a case of true allergy causing the skin disease. Although an IgE-mediated food allergy may contribute to the symptoms of atopic dermatitis in infants and young children, it is largely independent of the allergic factors among older children and adults.

A marked increase in allergic reactions has been noted with exposure to water-soluble proteins in latex products (e.g., rubber gloves, dental dams, condoms, tubing for respiratory equipment, catheters, and enema tips with inflatable latex cuffs). This is particularly true among medical personnel, patients exposed to latex, and children with spina bifida and urogenital birth defects.

There are two major kinds of allergy syndromes. Environmental allergies are triggered by inhalants or chemicals. Food allergies are triggered by your body's response to the proteins in certain foods.

Environmental Allergies

Hay fever is the most common environmental allergy syndrome, triggered by airborne pollens and mold spores. Hay fever is usually seasonal. During the spring and fall, people with hay fever experience increased symptoms of sneezing, congestion, and runny nose; they may also experience itchiness in the nose, roof of the mouth, throat, eyes, and ears, depending on where they live in the country and the exact allergen involved.

Common Environmental Allergic Substances
  Pollen (such as ragweed)
  Grasses
  Chemical fumes
  Cigarette smoke
  Aerosols
  Mold and mildew
  Perfumes
  Pet dander
  Smoke from BBQs, open fires, leaf burning
  Air pollution

Pollens are the tiny, egg-shaped male cells of flowering plants. These microscopic, powdery granules are necessary for plant fertilization. The average pollen particle is less than the width of a human hair. Pollens from plants with bright flowers, such as roses, usually do not trigger allergies. On the other hand, many trees, grasses, and low-growing weeds have small, light, dry pollens that are well-suited for dissemination by wind currents. These are the pollens that produce allergy symptoms.

Seasonal allergic rhinitis in the early spring is often triggered by the pollens of such trees as oak, western red cedar, elm, birch, ash, hickory, poplar, sycamore, maple, cypress, and walnut. In the late spring and early summer, pollinating grasses—including timothy, bermuda, orchard, sweet vernal, red top, and some bluegrasses—often trigger symptoms.

In addition to ragweed—the pollen most responsible for late summer and fall hay fever in North America—other weeds can trigger allergic rhinitis symptoms. These weeds include sagebrush, pigweed, tumbleweed, Russian thistle, and cockleweed. The period of pollination for these plants does not vary greatly from year to year. However, weather conditions can affect the amount of pollen in the air at any given time. The pollinating season starts later in the spring the farther north one goes.

Food Allergies

The incidence of food allergies has increased in the last fifteen years. This is probably due to a variety of factors, including earlier weaning and the introduction of solid foods to infants, genetic manipulation of plants resulting in foods that have a greater chance of cross-reacting with normal tissue, and an overall increase in the amount of pollutants in the air, soil, and food.

The most common allergic skin reaction to a food is hives. Hives are red, very itchy, swollen areas of the skin that may arise suddenly and leave quickly. They often appear in clusters, with new clusters appearing as other areas clear. Hives may occur alone, or be accompanied by other symptoms, such as swelling of the lips, tongue, and face. Food intolerance has been found to be responsible for the symptoms of some patients with irritable bowel syndrome. Preliminary information suggests that the same phenomenon may take place occasionally in patients with chronic ulcerative colitis. The first manifestation may be eczema, alone or in association with gastrointestinal symptoms. By the end of the first year, dermatitis usually has lessened and allergic respiratory symptoms may develop. Asthma and allergic rhinitis can be aggravated by allergy to foods.

Symptoms of food allergies may include a tingling sensation in the mouth, swelling of the tongue and throat, difficulty breathing, hives, vomiting, abdominal cramps, and diarrhea. These reactions may be accompanied by a drop in blood pressure and a loss of consciousness, which could lead to death. Symptoms typically appear within minutes to two hours after the person has eaten the food to which he or she is allergic.

The genetic predisposition to food allergies is well documented. In households where both parents are allergic, 67 percent of the offspring are allergic. Where one parent is allergic, 33 percent of the offspring are allergic. Immunologically produced food reactions result from the reaction of the food substance with sensitized IgE antibodies located on circulating mast cells. This leads to immediate hypersensitivity, so called because most of the symptoms develop within thirty to ninety minutes of ingesting the offending food. These symptoms include the well-known anaphylaxis symptoms of allergy—bronchial congestion and asthma, hives and eczema, headaches, loss of memory, and spaciness. (These reactions are caused by immune reactions, as opposed to other causes, such as inadequate stomach acid or esophageal reflux.)

Other conditions commonly associated with food allergies include such diverse problems as low back pain, bed-wetting, chronic bladder infections, canker sores, middle ear infections, asthma, acne, headache, and duodenal ulcers. Some of the common physical signs of allergy are dark circles or puffiness under the eyes, horizontal creases in the lower eyelid, swollen glands, and fluid retention.

However, the majority of so-called allergies are actually intolerances. Often, patients will come to my clinic complaining of allergies when technically they have intolerances or hypersensitivities. What is the difference? Simply put, a true allergy involves the activation of the IgE antibodies, whereas an intolerance does not. However, this doesn't mean that an intolerance is less serious or that it doesn't involve an immune reaction. For example, the problem some people have digesting the lactose in milk is not due to a lactose *allergy*. Rather, these individuals lack the specific enzyme needed to break it down. They are lactose *intolerant*.

The Role of Dietary Lectins

Most people have more to fear from hidden lectins entering their systems than from food allergies. Lectins are proteins in many foods that can bind to sugars (including blood type antigens) and cause cell damage.

According to the *British Journal of Nutrition*, which published a recent review of the subject, evidence exists that dietary lectins play a significant role in autoimmune and inflammatory diseases. The study seemed to indicate that interaction between dietary lectins and the cells lining the intestines may unnecessarily "rev up" the immune system and activate autoantibodies. Several dietary lectins, including those in peas and peanuts, have been shown to increase immunoglobulin A (IgA). IgA is the antibody most involved in the health of the digestive system. It is the main antibody in a variety of secretions such as saliva, milk, and the mucus lining the airways and digestive tract. Two common components of wheat, gliandin and gluten, have also been shown in repeated studies to increase the production of IgA.

Dietary lectins have also been shown to induce the production of interleukin-4, which in turn activates IgE. This may explain why one of the more common benefits reported by those who follow the Blood Type Diet is a lessening of allergic manifestations, sinusitis, and asthma. Many bacteria use lectins to attach to host tissue, and these lectins are some of the more highly allergenic parts of the organism. Many food lectins trigger IgE, including the lectins found in bananas, chestnuts, and avocados. They are all implicated in what has been termed "latex fruit allergies." Kiwi fruit lectins can also trigger IgE.

Lectins from peas, broad beans, lentils, jack beans, soy beans, peanuts, and wheat germ have been shown to bind directly with IgE and initiate the release of histamine, which can produce a feeling of spaciness, a condition characterized by an inability to focus and concentrate.

One of the most damaging effects of dietary lectins is a condition known as leaky gut syndrome. This occurs when partially digested proteins cross the intestinal barrier and are absorbed into the bloodstream. The mucus lining of the intestine consists of helpful bacteria and good yeasts that break down the food into substances that are used beneficially by the body's systems. When the composition of this lining is disturbed, the intestinal walls can be damaged and become porous. Overwhelmed by the flood of foreign substances, the immune system overreacts, causing allergic reactions at the site of transfer, at distant sites, or systemically.

Food Allergies and Ear Infections
As many as two-thirds of all children under six years of age suffer from chronic ear infections, accounting for half of all visits to pediatricians. Most of these children have allergies to both environmental and food-based particles.

Several studies have shown that the ear fluids of children with a history of chronic ear infections lack specific chemicals called complement, which are needed to attack and destroy the bacteria. One study showed that a crucial serum lectin known as mannose-binding protein is completely absent in the ear fluid of children with chronic infections. This lectin apparently binds to mannose sugars on the surface of the bacteria and agglutinates them, allowing for their efficient collection and removal. Both of these important immune system factors eventually do develop in sufficient quantities. This explains why the frequency of ear infections tends to gradually lessen as the children grow older.

Ear infections are terribly painful for a child. Most of these infections are a backup of noxious fluids and gasses into the middle ear because of an obstructed connecting pipe, the Eustachian tube. This tube can become swollen because of allergic reactions, weakness in the tissues surrounding it, or infections.

An often ignored risk factor for ear infections is food allergy or intolerance. The majority of children treated at my clinic for chronic ear infections are helped simply by eliminating allergic substances or reactive lectins from their diets.

Sinusitis

Sinusitis, a chronic inflammation of the nasal sinuses, usually begins with a cold. However, people with allergies seem to be predisposed to developing sinusitis because the inflammation of the sinuses and nasal mucus lining caused by allergies prevents the sinus cavities from clearing accumulated infection-creating bacteria.

Most people with chronic sinusitis have more than one factor that predisposes them to infection. Chronic sinusitis sufferers find that damp weather, especially in northern temperate climates, as well as pollutants in the air and pollutants and mold in buildings, affects them adversely. Some people who are allergic to fungi can develop a condition called allergic fungal sinusitis.

You might develop chronic sinusitis if you have an immune deficiency disease or an abnormality in the way mucus travels through your respiratory system (e.g., if you have immune deficiency, HIV infection, or cystic fibrosis). In addition, if you suffer from severe asthma, nasal polyps (small growths in the nose), or a severe asthmatic response to aspirin (or aspirinlike medicines, such as ibuprofen), you might develop chronic sinusitis.

Scientific studies have shown a close relationship between having allergic rhinitis and chronic sinusitis. Research suggests that up to 80 percent of adults with chronic sinusitis also have allergic rhinitis. There is also an association between asthma and sinusitis. Some researchers think that as many as 75 percent of people with asthma also get sinusitis.

Asthma

Asthma is most common in children under ten years old and is twice as common in males. Not everyone with allergies has asthma, but most people with asthma have some form of allergy.

There are two kinds of asthma:

Extrinsic asthma: Also called atopic asthma, this is considered to be IgE-mediated. Attacks are mostly initiated by exposure to allergens: dust, molds, pollens, animal dander, and foods.

Intrinsic asthma: This form does not seem related to an antigen-antibody complex. Rather, the bronchial reaction is due to other factors, such as cold air, exercise, infection, emotional upset, and irritating inhalants.

Most asthma sufferers have a mixture of the two kinds, although extrinsic asthma is more common in infants and children.

The signs and symptoms of asthma vary widely. Some asthmatics have symptoms all of the time, whereas others have asymptomatic (meaning they are doing just fine, thank you) periods followed by severe episodes. Mild symptoms may include slight coughing followed by minor wheezing. Sometimes symptoms start with light coughing and progress into severe coughing, often accompanied by extreme difficulty in breathing. In children, a tightening sensation over the anterior neck or upper chest is an early sign of an impending attack. Often a certain stressor—such as exercise or breathing cold air or some noxious agent—may initiate the onset of an attack. Over a long period of time, asthma can wear out the body's adrenal and immune functions, causing severe fatigue and susceptibility to infection.

Diagnosing Allergies

Diagnosing allergies can seem like a complex business. I've had patients come to my clinic after undergoing months of being pricked, prodded, and tested with potentially offending substances—all in the interests of determining precisely which substances in food or the environment provoke allergic reactions. I consider most allergy testing to be a waste of time and money.

The problem with most standard allergy testing, such as the RAST test, is that it doesn't account for the wide range of reactions that occur when people are hypersensitive to or intolerant of substances. For example, reactions to dietary lectins will not show up in standard tests. It is important to look beyond symptoms and IgE-mediated reactions to determine how a food or substance is affecting the entire physiology—the metabolism, immune system, and digestive system. Balancing the system is of paramount importance.

After many years of clinical observation, I have discovered that for most of my patients, the Blood Type Diet is the most effective starting point in their battle against allergic reactions.

The Blood Type–Allergy Connection

NATURE HAS ENDOWED OUR IMMUNE SYSTEMS WITH VERY sophisticated methods to determine if a substance in the body is foreign or not. One method involves looking for chemical markers called antigens, which are found on the cells of our bodies and on most other living things. Any substance could be an antigen; the only requirement is that it be unique enough to allow the immune system an opportunity to determine if it is "self" or "non-self."

All life forms, from the simplest virus to humans, have unique antigens that form a part of their chemical fingerprint. Among the many antigens in your body is one that determines blood type. When your immune system is attempting to identify a suspicious character, one of the first things it looks for is your blood type antigen.

Each blood type is determined by the presence or absence of an antigen with a unique chemical structure composed of long chains of a repeating sugar called fucose, which by itself forms the O antigen of Blood Type O. Fucose also serves as the base for the other blood types.

Blood Type A is composed of fucose, plus a sugar named N-acetyl galactosamine. Blood Type B is fucose, plus a different sugar named D-galactosamine. Blood Type AB is fucose, plus N-acetyl galactosamine, plus D-galactosamine.

Each blood type antigen creates opposing antibodies to other blood type antigens. These anti–blood type antibodies are often called isohemagglutinins because they are made throughout life and are IgM antibodies, so they can agglutinate antigens directly. These are very powerful antibodies! The best known role of the isohemagglutinins is seen in the transfusion reaction. This occurs when someone is inadvertently given the wrong blood type during a transfusion. This process can be very serious. A person who receives an incompatible blood transfusion may experience fever, shaking, chills, shortness of

Blood Type Antigens and Antibodies

BLOOD TYPE	ANTIGEN	ANTIBODIES
O	None—or "zero"— (fucose)	You produce antibodies to Blood Types A, B, and AB. You can only receive Type O blood, but you can donate blood to all types. Because of this, Type O is often referred to as the universal donor. However, you consider all things in nature that are A-like or B-like foreign.
A	A	You produce antibodies to Blood Type B. You can receive blood from Blood Types O and A, but you consider all things in nature that are B-like foreign.
B	B	You produce antibodies to Blood Type A. You can receive blood from Blood Types O and B, but you consider all things in nature that are A-like foreign.
AB	A and B	Because both A and B antigens are present in your red blood cells, you don't carry antibodies for either. You can receive blood from Blood Types O, A, B, and AB. Because of this, Blood Type AB is often called the universal receiver.

breath, hives, and nausea. Shock, kidney failure, or blood coagulation can ensue, and even death may occur, although rare.

Many substances, such as bacteria, viruses, parasites, and some foods, actually resemble foreign blood type antigens, and it is the job of your blood type antibodies to recognize these intruders and target them for removal.

About ten years ago, I measured the levels of these anti–blood type antibodies in several people with a variety of physical ailments. Not surprisingly, in several illnesses characterized by autoimmune dysfunction or excess inflammation, the levels of these antibodies were often found to be sky high. This was especially true in conditions associated with a hyperactive immune or inflammatory response. They included rheumatoid arthritis, chronic ear infection, Crohn's disease, asthma, eczema, and hives. Since they serve to protect against infection, it is not surprising that the levels of anti–blood type antibodies can increase in times of acute infection.

Secretors and Non-Secretors

ALTHOUGH EVERYONE CARRIES a blood type antigen on their blood cells, about 80 percent of the population also secretes blood type antigens into body fluids, such as saliva, mucus, and sperm. These people are called secretors. The approximately 20 percent of the population that does not secrete blood type antigens into body fluids are called non-secretors. Being a secretor is independent of your ABO group, thus there are both Type O secretors and Type O non-secretors.

Since blood type antigens are crucial to the integrity of the gut immune defense, being unable to secrete them into body fluids can place non-secretors at a disadvantage. In general, non-secretors are far more likely to suffer from immune diseases than secretors, especially when the disease is provoked by an infectious organism. Non-secretors also have genetically induced difficulties removing immune complexes from their tissues, provoking inflammatory conditions.

Blood Type–Specific Dietary Lectins

WHILE SOME LECTINS react with the tissues of all blood types, many lectins are blood type–specific, in that they show a clear preference for one kind of sugar over another and mechanically fit the antigen of one blood type or another. This blood type specificity results in their attaching to the antigen of a preferred blood type, while leaving other blood type antigens completely undisturbed. At the cellular level, a common effect of lectins is to provoke the sugars on the surface of one cell to cross-link with those of another, effectively causing the cells to stick together and agglutinate. Not all lectins cause agglutination; many bacteria have lectinlike receptors that they use to attach to the cells of their host. Other lectins, called mitogens, cause a proliferation of certain cells of the immune system. But, in the most basic sense, lectins make things stick to other things.

Your Blood Type Susceptibility

ALL BLOOD TYPES can suffer from allergies. However, there are variations in susceptibility and in the specific triggers.

Blood Type O

Blood Type O is more prone to inflammation than the other blood types and tends to have higher levels of IgE and IgA. This vulnerability is possibly related to the fucose sugar that acts as its blood type antigen. Fucose sugars are known to serve as adhesion molecules for selectins, allowing the hyperactive migration of white blood cells from the bloodstream into areas of infection, which in turn causes inflammation. Studies have shown that Blood Type O individuals tend to dramatically increase the levels of their anti-A and anti-B antibodies during infections.

Blood Type O individuals are more likely to be asthma sufferers, and even hay fever, the bane of so many, appears to be specific to Type O blood. A wide range of pollens contains lectins that stimulate the release of the powerful histamines that lead to the common allergy symptoms. Many food lectins, especially wheat, interact with IgE antibodies found in Type O blood. These antibodies stimulate white blood cells called basophiles to release not only histamines but also other powerful chemical allergens called kinins. These can cause severe allergic reactions, swelling the tissues of the throat and constricting the lungs. Type Os who eliminate wheat from their diets often relieve many of their allergy symptoms, such as sneezing, respiratory problems, snoring, or persistent digestive disorders.

Digestively, Blood Type O's extreme sensitivity to the lectins in wheat and corn makes them more vulnerable to inflammatory conditions such as leaky gut syndrome and increases their susceptibility to irritable bowel syndrome and Crohn's disease.

According to research, non-secretor status plays a prominent role in Blood Type O's susceptibility to allergies.

Blood Type A

There are several pathways to allergies for Blood Type A. One is the tendency to produce high levels of selectins in response to infection or injury. Overproduction of selectins, E-selectin in particular, produces a hyperactive or inflammatory response. Several components of the diet are known to influence selectin levels. High animal protein diets further increase E-selectin, while a diet featuring more soy protein significantly lowers selectin levels. One important component of soy, the isoflavone genestein, inhibits enzymes necessary to increase selectins and other vascular adhesion molecules.

Blood Type A children (or even children with Blood Type A mothers) are more prone to develop ear infections. In general, Blood Type A children have about a 50 percent higher rate of infection. Strains of bacteria most likely to cause ear infections have a very strong preference for the Blood Type A antigen. This is especially true for non-secretors. A contributory trigger is Blood Type A's tendency to produce copious amounts of mucus, which can exacerbate ear infections and certain respiratory conditions. In Blood Type A children, dairy products are often the culprit in excessive mucus production.

Blood Type A also has a predisposition to bronchial asthma in childhood, and Type A individuals are generally more asthmatic.

Digestively, Blood Type A individuals who consume too much animal protein—especially red meat—tend to suffer from leaky gut syndrome. Type As have low levels of digestive enzymes, making it difficult for them to digest meat. The result is undigested proteins that take far too long to transit the intestines and eliminate from the system.

Blood Type B

Overall, Blood Type B is associated with greater severity of chronic inflammatory diseases of the lungs, including bronchial asthma and pollinosis. Research shows that Blood Type B has a higher susceptibility to grass pollen hay fever than do the other blood types. Often the trigger is dietary, as Blood Type B individuals have intense sensitivities to a diverse number of lectins, such as those found in chicken, corn, wheat, soy, and peanuts.

Blood Type B's susceptibility to viral infection appears to be related to their sensitivity to a class of agglutinins called galectins, found in all animals but most notably found in chicken meat. Galectins are considered a type of "internal lectin" made by higher animals and used for a variety of specialized functions, especially within the liver. They bind several different galactose-antigens, and it is probably for this reason that chicken seems to agglutinate the cells of Blood Types B and AB. Several galectins are known to involve themselves in the inflammatory process. For example, urinary tract infections, to which Blood Type B individuals are prone, are known triggers for subsequent inflammatory diseases.

Blood Type AB

Blood Type AB has the highest resistance to respiratory allergies of all the blood types. However, Blood Type AB is somewhat susceptible to the conditions related to both the A and B antigens. Like Blood Type A,

Type AB has a tendency toward overstimulation of selectins on the blood vessel walls, which allows excessive white blood cell migration into the tissues and triggers inflammation. Blood Type AB also shares the Type A tendency for overproduction of mucus and somewhat lower than normal levels of stomach acid. Like Blood Type B, Type AB is susceptible to viral and bacterial infections, and these in turn can trigger autoimmune inflammatory responses, often through inactivating complement or blocking the liver's ability to detoxify normal metabolic waste products.

More than the other blood types, Blood Type AB is affected by diminished activity of natural killer (NK) cells. NK cells are a subset of T-lymphocytes, which function as a first line of defense against infection.

Non-Secretors

Regardless of blood type, being non-secretor heightens the risk of allergies and other inflammatory conditions. Research has revealed the following about non-secretors:

- Non-secretors are more prone to generalized inflammation and have higher levels of IgE than secretors.
- Non-secretors have an increased prevalence of a variety of autoimmune diseases.
- IgA levels are significantly lower in non-secretors than in secretors. The lower levels of IgA cannot prevent microorganisms from gaining access to the bloodstream from the oral cavity and digestive tract.
- Non-secretors tend to have a higher incidence of asthma.
- Non-secretors tend to have a higher incidence of infection and compromised immunity.

Since secretor status is a critical factor in preventing and treating allergies, the individualized Blood Type Diet plans include variations based on secretor status. An at-home blood-typing kit is available through our Web site at www.dadamo.com.

For more information about health factors associated with your secretor status, refer to *Live Right 4 Your Type* and *The Complete Blood Type Encyclopedia*. Extensive study references related to the blood type specificities of inflammatory disease are available for review on our Web site.

THREE

Fighting Allergies with Conventional and Blood Type Therapies

THE CONVENTIONAL ALLERGY TREATMENTS THAT MOST people are familiar with emphasize avoidance of offending allergens and alleviating symptoms. Obviously, it makes sense to avoid substances that provoke allergic reactions. However, the regular use of antihistamines, antibiotics, antacids, and other medications fails to address the underlying mechanisms of illness, and overuse can ultimately be counterproductive.

Scientific studies have verified that, while antihistamines and aspirin can temporarily relieve discomfort, their use may prolong the course of the attack. Fever and inflammation are not just symptoms, but also healing mechanisms. Inflammation is an increase in blood flow to an area, and fever is part of the body's way of killing harmful organisms. However, taking aspirin or an antihistamine combats these efforts by the body to heal itself. Over time, these medications can weaken the immune system. For example, histamine is critical for the proper binding of NK cells to their potential targets, so the chronic use of antihistamines might account for some of the observed reduction in NK activity in people with severe allergies.

The same is true with antibiotics. Antibiotics are the treatment of choice for childhood ear infections, but there is growing worry that the overuse of antibiotics is making the bacteria that cause ear infections—and more serious ailments—resistant to the drugs. Why do antibiotics stop working? A baby's first ear infection is typically treated with a mild antibiotic such as amoxicillin. With the child's next ear infection, amoxicillin is given again. Eventually, the ever more resistant infection returns, and amoxicillin is no longer effective. The escalation phenomenon—the process of using stronger and stronger drugs, and ever more invasive treatments—has begun. It's a vicious cycle that can cause long-term damage.

Most people see no harm in taking antacids to treat gastric discomfort. However, taking antacid medications, which affect acid secretion or neutralize the pH within the stomach, may be setting up a situation where harmless food proteins turn into potential allergens. Gastric digestion depends on the presence of acid and pepsin, a protein-degrading enzyme activated at high acidic levels. However, elevation of pH levels hinders pepsin secretion, which hampers protein digestion.

It is doubtful that drug therapy alone can successfully cure inflammatory bowel disease. Drug therapy for inflammatory bowel disease strikes me as similar to policing a bad neighborhood. Certainly the police are needed to root out the criminals and attempt to keep the streets safe, but the neighborhood will never actually become stable—and, in the case of inflammatory bowel disease, healthy—unless the underlying causes of the problem are dealt with.

The ultimate goal of any treatment must go beyond just getting over the latest bout with illness. That's where the Blood Type Diet comes in. If you are being treated for allergies, sinusitis, asthma, or related conditions, talk to your physician about incorporating these long-term strategies into your program.

Fighting Allergies with the Blood Type Diet

THE BLOOD TYPE DIET and its related lifestyle/supplement strategies can help you fight allergies by:

Attacking the underlying causes of allergies The Blood Type Diet promotes a healthy immune system, reducing the potential for infections that can trigger the inflammatory process.

Relieving allergy symptoms Adhering to the diet that is right for your blood type is a proven way to relieve symptoms by eliminating immunoreactive lectins that trigger allergic responses.

Alleviating the need for allergy medications Antihistamines, antacids, antibiotics, corticosteroids, and other medications can have damaging side effects. Frequently, those who follow the Blood Type Diet experience major relief of symptoms and no longer need these medications. (A caveat: Never discontinue prescription medications without consulting your physician.)

Establishing overall health and fitness The Blood Type Diet utilizes the best of naturopathic medicine, combined with individualized diet, exercise, and lifestyle strategies that support maximum health. The Blood Type Diet is nutritionally tailored to emphasize foods that support digestive, immune, and metabolic balance.

ARE YOU READY TO BEGIN? Find your blood type section, and we'll place you on the right diet to fight allergies.

PART II

Individualized Blood Type Plans

FOUR

Blood Type

BLOOD TYPE O DIET OUTCOME: CUDDLING WITH THE CAT

"In the first week I just eliminated the 'avoids,' and immediately my sinuses drained for that week. Although I've had major allergies to animals all my life, I no longer have any allergic reaction to the cat. Finally, for the first time ever, I'm not sneezing anymore."

BLOOD TYPE O DIET OUTCOME: LIFELONG ALLERGIES DISAPPEAR

"The grass/pollen allergies that I have had since age twelve have completely disappeared. I do not react to mosquito or flea bites, either. I have purposely gone off the diet, and the allergies have reappeared in two to four hours. My energy has at least doubled. These results began to appear only two weeks into the diet."

BLOOD TYPE O DIET OUTCOME: TASTE AND SMELL RESTORED

"I had no sense of taste or smell for eight years, unless I took steroids, which I did once or twice a year. I had asthma and chronic sinusitis, and often could breathe only through my mouth. I tried all the conventional strategies— surgery for nasal polyps, antihistamines, asthma medications, OTC reme- dies, allergy shots, and probably every antibiotic known to medical science.

I decided to follow the Blood Type Diet recommendations to the letter—no more wheat products at all, no more potatoes, no more dairy, and all the other little no-no's—e.g., Brussels sprouts. I can't believe how well the diet worked. My senses of taste and smell have been perfect! The asthma is all gone, and I can breathe like a normal person."

Self-reported outcomes from the Blood Type Diet Web site (www.dadamo.com)

Blood Type O: The Foods

THE BLOOD TYPE O Allergy Diet is specifically adapted for the prevention and management of allergic conditions. In particular, it addresses Type O's unique susceptibilities, including a tendency to develop inflammatory conditions and sensitivities to the lectins in many foods. A new category, **Super Beneficial,** highlights powerful disease-fighting foods for Blood Type O. The **Neutral** category has also been adjusted to de-emphasize foods that are less advantageous for you. Foods designated **Neutral: Allowed Infrequently** should be severely minimized or eliminated entirely.

Your secretor status can influence your ability to fully digest and metabolize certain foods, so various adjustments in the values are made for non-secretors. If you do not know your secretor type, the odds are that you can safely use the values given for secretors. The majority of the population (almost 80 percent) are secretors. However, I urge you to get tested, since the variations are important for non-secretors who want to maximize the effectiveness of the Blood Type Diet. To find out how to get tested, visit our Web site (www.dadamo.com).

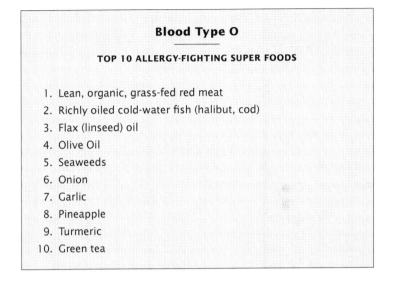

Blood Type O
_____

TOP 10 ALLERGY-FIGHTING SUPER FOODS

1. Lean, organic, grass-fed red meat
2. Richly oiled cold-water fish (halibut, cod)
3. Flax (linseed) oil
4. Olive Oil
5. Seaweeds
6. Onion
7. Garlic
8. Pineapple
9. Turmeric
10. Green tea

The food charts are divided into three sections. The top of the chart suggests the average portion size and quantity per week or day, according to secretor status. These recommendations do *not* apply to the category **Neutral: Allowed Infrequently;** those foods should be eaten rarely, if at all. The charts also indicate differences in frequency for some foods based on ethnic heritage. It has been my experience that this factor has an impact upon the individual's ability to fully digest certain foods. For the purposes of blood type food choices, persons of Hispanic heritage should follow the guidelines for Caucasians, and American Native peoples should follow the guidelines for Asians.

The middle section of the chart gives the food values. The bottom section lists variations based on secretor status.

For your convenience, we have included a number of product names (Ezekiel 4:9 bread, Worcestershire sauce, etc.). However, keep in mind that commercial formulations vary among brands and regions. Even though a product may be listed as acceptable for you, always check its ingredients. Some products may contain **Avoid** ingredients for your blood type. Of course, you may choose to make your own version of commercial products, such as bread and mayonnaise, using ingredients that suit your blood type. There are hundreds of delicious recipes for every blood type available on our Web site (www. dadamo.com) and in the book *Cook Right 4 Your Type: The Practical Kitchen Companion to* Eat Right 4 Your Type.

Meat/Poultry

Protein in the form of lean, organic meat is critical for Blood Type O and is the key to digestive health and immune function. This is even more important for non-secretors. High-quality animal protein is easily digested by Blood Type O, helping to ward off intestinal problems associated with allergies. Choose only the best quality (preferably free-range), chemical-, antibiotic-, and pesticide-free low-fat meats and poultry. Grass-fed cattle and buffalo are far superior to grain-fed.

BLOOD TYPE O: MEAT/POULTRY			
Portion: 4–6 oz (men); 2–5 oz (women and children)			
	African	Caucasian	Asian
Secretor	6–9	6–9	6–9
Non-Secretor	7–12	7–12	7–11
		Times per week	

SUPER BENEFICIAL	BENEFICIAL	NEUTRAL: Allowed Frequently	NEUTRAL: Allowed Infrequently	AVOID
Beef	Heart (calf)	Chicken		All commercially processed meats
Buffalo	Liver (calf)	Cornish hen		Bacon/ham/pork
Lamb	Mutton	Duck		Quail
	Sweetbreads	Goat		Turtle
	Veal	Goose		
	Venison	Grouse		
		Guinea hen		
		Horse		

SUPER BENEFICIAL	BENEFICIAL	NEUTRAL: Allowed Frequently	NEUTRAL: Allowed Infrequently	AVOID
		Ostrich		
		Partridge		
		Pheasant		
		Rabbit		
		Squab		
		Squirrel		
		Turkey		

Special Variants: *Non-Secretor* BENEFICIAL: ostrich, partridge, pheasant, rabbit, squab; NEUTRAL (Allowed Frequently): lamb, liver (calf), quail, turtle.

Fish/Seafood

Fish and seafood represent a secondary source of high-quality protein for Blood Type O. In particular, richly oiled cold-water fish like cod, halibut, red snapper, and trout are SUPER BENEFICIAL for Blood Type O. These fish contain beneficial omega-3 fatty acids, such as docosahexaenoic acid (DHA) and eicosapentaenoic acid (EPA), and are considered anti-inflammatory; they reduce the effects of inflammatory fats.

BLOOD TYPE O: FISH/SEAFOOD			
Portion: 4–6 oz (men); 2–5 oz (women and children)			
	African	Caucasian	Asian
Secretor	2–4	3–5	2–5
Non-Secretor	2–5	4–5	4–5
		Times per week	

SUPER BENEFICIAL	BENEFICIAL	NEUTRAL: Allowed Frequently	NEUTRAL: Allowed Infrequently	AVOID
Cod	Bass (all)	Beluga	Anchovy	Abalone
Halibut	Perch (all)	Bluefish	Crab	Barracuda
Red snapper	Pike	Bullhead	Eel	Catfish
	Shad	Butterfish	Flounder	Conch

SUPER BENEFICIAL	BENEFICIAL	NEUTRAL: Allowed Frequently	NEUTRAL: Allowed Infrequently	AVOID
Trout (rainbow)	Sole (except gray) Sturgeon Swordfish Tilefish Yellowtail	Carp Caviar (sturgeon) Chub Clam Croaker Cusk Drum Haddock Hake Halfmoon fish Harvest fish Herring (fresh) Lobster Mackerel Mahi-mahi Monkfish Mullet Opaleye Orange roughy Oyster Parrot fish Pickerel Pompano Porgy Rosefish Sailfish Salmon Sardine	Gray sole Grouper Mussel Whitefish	Frog Herring (pickled/ smoked) Muskel- lunge Octopus Pollock Salmon (smoked) Salmon roe Squid (calamari)

SUPER BENEFICIAL	BENEFICIAL	NEUTRAL: Allowed Frequently	NEUTRAL: Allowed Infrequently	AVOID
		Scallop		
		Scrod		
		Shark		
		Shrimp		
		Smelt		
		Snail (*Helix pomatia/* escargot)		
		Sucker		
		Sunfish		
		Tilapia		
		Trout (brook/ sea)		
		Tuna		
		Weakfish		
		Whiting		

Special Variants: *Non-Secretor* BENEFICIAL: hake, herring (fresh), mackerel, sardine; NEUTRAL (Allowed Frequently): bass, catfish, halibut, red snapper, salmon roe; AVOID: anchovy, crab, mussel.

Dairy/Eggs

Most dairy foods should be avoided by Blood Type O. They are poorly digested and metabolized and often trigger or enhance allergic reactions. Ghee (clarified butter) is one exception because it's a good source of butyrate, which supports Blood Type O intestinal health. Eggs can be consumed in moderation, but should be limited by allergy sufferers. Do your best to find eggs and dairy products—if you must use them—that are both hormone-free and organic.

BLOOD TYPE O: EGGS

Portion: 1 egg

	African	Caucasian	Asian
Secretor	1–4	3–6	3–4
Non-Secretor	2–5	3–6	3–4
		Times per week	

BLOOD TYPE O: MILK AND YOGURT

Portion: 4–6 oz (men); 2–5 oz (women and children)

	African	Caucasian	Asian
Secretor	0–1	0–3	0–2
Non-Secretor	0	0–2	0–3
		Times per week	

BLOOD TYPE O: CHEESE

Portion: 3 oz (men); 2 oz (women and children)

	African	Caucasian	Asian
Secretor	0–1	0–2	0–1
Non-Secretor	0	0–1	0
		Times per week	

SUPER BENEFICIAL	BENEFICIAL	NEUTRAL: Allowed Frequently	NEUTRAL: Allowed Infrequently	AVOID
	Ghee (clarified butter)	Egg (chicken/ duck)	Butter Farmer cheese Feta Goat cheese Mozzarella	American cheese Blue cheese Brie Buttermilk Camembert Casein Cheddar Colby Cottage cheese

SUPER BENEFICIAL	BENEFICIAL	NEUTRAL: Allowed Frequently	NEUTRAL: Allowed Infrequently	AVOID
				Cream cheese
				Edam
				Egg (goose/ quail)
				Emmenthal
				Gouda
				Gruyère
				Half-and- half
				Ice cream
				Jarlsberg
				Kefir
				Milk (cow/ goat)
				Monterey Jack
				Muenster
				Neufchâtel
				Paneer
				Parmesan
				Provolone
				Quark
				Ricotta
				Sherbet
				Sour cream
				String cheese
				Swiss cheese
				Whey
				Yogurt

Special Variants: *Non-Secretor* NEUTRAL (Allowed Frequently): Egg (goose/quail); AVOID: farmer cheese, feta, goat cheese, mozzarella.

Oils

Olive oil, a monounsaturated oil, is SUPER BENEFICIAL for Blood Type O. Constituents in olive oil, such as flavonoids, squalenes, and polyphenols, act as powerful antioxidants. It should be used as the primary cooking oil. Also SUPER BENEFICIAL is flax (linseed) oil, high in alpha-linolenic acid, which has anti-inflammatory properties. Be aware that some oils are high in omega-6 fatty acids, which can stimulate an inflammatory response. These include corn, cottonseed, peanut, and safflower oils. Secretors have a bit of an edge over non-secretors in digesting oils and probably benefit a bit more from their consumption.

BLOOD TYPE O: OILS			
Portion: 1 tblsp			
	African	Caucasian	Asian
Secretor	3–8	4–8	5–8
Non-Secretor	1–7	3–5	3–6
	Times per week		

SUPER BENEFICIAL	BENEFICIAL	NEUTRAL: Allowed Frequently	NEUTRAL: Allowed Infrequently	AVOID
Flax (linseed) Olive		Almond Black currant seed Borage seed Cod liver Sesame Walnut	Canola	Castor Coconut Corn Cottonseed Evening primrose Peanut Safflower Soy Sunflower Wheat germ

Special Variants: *Non-Secretor:* BENEFICIAL: almond, walnut; NEUTRAL (Allowed Frequently): coconut, flax (linseed); AVOID: borage, canola, cod liver.

Nuts/Seeds

Raw flax seeds are helpful for a strong immune system, providing beneficial omega-3 fatty acids. Walnuts are also SUPER BENEFICIAL. They are one of the best plant sources of omega-3 fatty acids. Walnuts are also highly effective in inhibiting gastrointestinal toxicity. Overall, however, you should limit your intake of nuts and seeds, especially if you have allergies. Many nuts and seeds, including beechnuts, sunflower seeds, and chestnuts, possess lectin or other immune reactivity for Blood Type O.

BLOOD TYPE O: NUTS/SEEDS			
Portion: Whole (handful); Nut Butters (2 tblsp)			
	African	Caucasian	Asian
Secretor	2–5	2–5	2–4
Non-Secretor	5–7	5–7	5–7
			Times per week

SUPER BENEFICIAL	BENEFICIAL	NEUTRAL: Allowed Frequently	NEUTRAL: Allowed Infrequently	AVOID
Flax Walnut (black/ English)	Pumpkin seed	Almond Almond butter Almond cheese Almond milk Butternut Filbert (hazelnut) Hickory Macadamia Pecan Pignolia (pine nut)	Safflower seed Sesame butter (tahini) Sesame seed	Beechnut Brazil nut Cashew Chestnut Litchi Peanut Peanut butter Pistachio Poppy seed Sunflower butter Sunflower seed

Special Variants: *Non-Secretor* NEUTRAL (Allowed Frequently): flax (linseed); AVOID: almond cheese, almond milk, safflower seed.

Beans/Legumes

Essentially carnivores when it comes to protein requirements, Blood Type Os should minimize consumption of beans and legumes. Many of them, such as lentils, contain pro-inflammatory lectins. Given the choice, get your protein from animal foods.

BLOOD TYPE O: BEANS/LEGUMES			
Portion: 1 cup (cooked)			
	African	Caucasian	Asian
Secretor	1–3	1–3	2–4
Non-Secretor	0–2	0–3	2–4
		Times per week	

SUPER BENEFICIAL	BENEFICIAL	NEUTRAL: Allowed Frequently	NEUTRAL: Allowed Infrequently	AVOID
	Adzuki bean	Black bean	Soy milk	Copper bean
	Bean (green/ snap/ string)	Cannellini bean		Kidney bean
		Garbanzo (chick-pea)		Lentil (all)
	Black-eyed pea			Navy bean
	Fava (broad) bean	Jicama bean		Pinto bean
	Northern bean	Lima bean		Tamarind bean
		Mung bean/ sprouts		
		Pea (green/ pod/ snow)		
		Soy bean		
		Soy cheese		

SUPER BENEFICIAL	BENEFICIAL	NEUTRAL: Allowed Frequently	NEUTRAL: Allowed Infrequently	AVOID
		Soy, miso		
		Soy, tempeh		
		Soy, tofu		
		White bean		

Special Variants: *Non-Secretor* NEUTRAL (Allowed Frequently): adzuki bean, black-eyed pea, lentil (all), pinto bean; AVOID: fava (broad) bean, garbanzo (chickpea), soy (all).

Grains/Starches

Consumption of most grains and starches will exacerbate allergic and inflammatory conditions for Blood Type O. You do poorly on corn, wheat, sorghum, barley, and many of their by-products (sweeteners, etc.). In particular, the lectin in wheat produces gut inflammation and is the primary cause of celiac disease. Wheat is also a leading factor in the development of inflammatory conditions for Blood Type O. The exceptions are sprouted seed breads, such as Essene and Ezekiel 4:9, usually found in the freezer section of your health-food store. The gluten lectins, principally found in the seed coats, are destroyed in the sprouting process. Unlike many commercially sprouted breads, Essene and Ezekiel 4:9 are "live" foods, with many beneficial enzymes intact.

Non-secretors have even greater wheat sensitivity. Non-secretors should avoid oats, as well.

BLOOD TYPE O: GRAINS/STARCHES			
Portion: ½ cup dry (grains or pastas); 1 muffin; 2 slices of bread			
	African	Caucasian	Asian
Secretor	1–6	1–6	1–6
Non-Secretor	0–3	0–3	0–3
		Times per week	

SUPER BENEFICIAL	BENEFICIAL	NEUTRAL: Allowed Frequently	NEUTRAL: Allowed Infrequently	AVOID
	Essene bread (manna)	Amaranth	Buckwheat	Barley
		Ezekiel 4:9 bread	Millet	Cornmeal
		Kamut	Oat bran	Couscous
		Quinoa	Oat flour	Grits
		Spelt (whole)	Oatmeal	Popcorn
		Spelt flour/ products	Rice (whole)	Sorghum
		Tapioca	Rice (wild)	Wheat (refined/ unbleached)
		Teff	Rice cake	Wheat (semolina)
		100% sprouted grain products (except Essene)	Rice flour	Wheat (white flour)
			Rice milk	Wheat (whole)
			Rye (whole)	Wheat bran
			Rye flour/ products	Wheat germ
			Soba noodles (100% buck- wheat)	
			Soy flour/ products	

Special Variants: *Non-Secretor* AVOID: buckwheat, oat (all), soba noodles (100% buckwheat), soy flour/products, spelt (whole), spelt flour/products, tapioca.

Vegetables

Vegetables provide a rich source of antioxidants and fiber, and the right choices can help Blood Type O balance immune functions. Fucose-containing seaweeds are SUPER BENEFICIAL in blocking lectin activity. They serve as a food source for beneficial colon bacteria, thus reducing gut inflammation. Onions are high in quercetin, a flavonoid with potent anti-inflammatory properties. Sweet potatoes are rich in vitamins A and B_6, which stabilize immune function. Several vegetables are pro-inflammatory for Blood Type O and should be minimized or avoided. These include the so-called nightshade family—white potatoes, peppers, eggplant, and tomatoes.

An item's value also applies to its juice, unless otherwise noted.

BLOOD TYPE O: VEGETABLES			
Portion: 1 cup, prepared (cooked or raw)			
	African	Caucasian	Asian
Secretor Super/Beneficials	Unlimited	Unlimited	Unlimited
Secretor Neutrals	2–5	2–5	2–5
Non-Secretor Super/Beneficials	Unlimited	Unlimited	Unlimited
Non-Secretor Neutrals	2–3	2–3	2–3
			Times per day

SUPER BENEFICIAL	BENEFICIAL	NEUTRAL: Allowed Frequently	NEUTRAL: Allowed Infrequently	AVOID
Broccoli	Artichoke	Arugula	Brussels sprouts	Alfalfa sprouts
Collards	Beet	Asparagus	Cabbage	Aloe
Kale	Beet greens	Asparagus pea	Eggplant	Cauliflower
Onion (all)	Chicory	Bamboo shoot	Olive (Greek/ green/ Spanish)	Corn
Seaweeds	Dandelion	Bok choy	Peppers (all)	Cucumber
Spinach	Escarole	Carrot	Tomato	Leek
	Horse- radish	Celeriac	Yam	Mushroom (shiitake/ silver dollar)
	Kohlrabi	Celery		Mustard greens
	Lettuce (Romaine)	Chili pepper		Olive (black)
		Daikon radish		Potato

SUPER BENEFICIAL	BENEFICIAL	NEUTRAL: Allowed Frequently	NEUTRAL: Allowed Infrequently	AVOID
	Mushroom (abalone/ enoki/ maitake/ oyster/ porto-bello/ straw/ tree ear) Okra Parsnip Potato (sweet) Pumpkin Swiss chard Turnip	Endive Fennel Fiddlehead fern Garlic Lettuce (except Romaine) Poi Radicchio Radish/ sprouts Rappini (broccoli rabe) Rutabaga Scallion Shallot Squash Water chestnut Watercress Zucchini		

Special Variants: *Non-Secretor* BENEFICIAL: carrot, fiddlehead fern, garlic; NEU-TRAL (Allowed Frequently): lettuce (Romaine), mushroom (except shiitake), mustard greens, parsnip, potato (sweet), turnip; AVOID: Brussels sprouts, cabbage, egg-plant, olive (all), poi.

Fruits and Fruit Juices

Blood Type O should consume lots of fruits rich in antioxidants, vitamins, and fiber. SUPER BENEFICIAL are blueberries, cherries, and elderberries. Pineapple contains bromelain, a powerful enzyme that has an anti-inflammatory effect. Several citrus fruits, such as kiwi and oranges, are implicated in irritable bowel syndrome and contain O-reactive lectins.

An item's value also applies to its juices, unless otherwise noted.

BLOOD TYPE O: FRUITS AND FRUIT JUICES			
Portion: 1 cup			
	African	Caucasian	Asian
Secretor	2–4	3–5	3–5
Non-Secretor	1–3	1–3	1–3
			Times per day

SUPER BENEFICIAL	BENEFICIAL	NEUTRAL: Allowed Frequently	NEUTRAL: Allowed Infrequently	AVOID
Blueberry	Banana	Boysen-berry	Apple	Asian pear
Cherry	Fig (fresh/dried)	Breadfruit	Apricot	Avocado
Elderberry (dark blue/purple)	Guava	Canang melon	Currant	Bitter melon
Pineapple	Mango	Casaba melon	Date	Blackberry
	Plum	Christmas melon	Grape (all)	Cantaloupe
	Prune	Cranberry	Quince	Coconut
		Crenshaw melon	Raisin	Honeydew
		Dewberry	Star fruit (carambola)	Kiwi
		Goose-berry	Strawberry	Orange
		Grapefruit		Plantain
				Tangerine

SUPER BENEFICIAL	BENEFICIAL	NEUTRAL: Allowed Frequently	NEUTRAL: Allowed Infrequently	AVOID
		Kumquat		
		Lemon		
		Lime		
		Logan-berry		
		Mulberry		
		Musk-melon		
		Nectarine		
		Papaya		
		Peach		
		Pear		
		Persian melon		
		Persimmon		
		Pome-granate		
		Prickly pear		
		Raspberry		
		Sago palm		
		Spanish melon		
		Water-melon		
		Young-berry		

Special Variants: *Non-Secretor* BENEFICIAL: avocado, pomegranate, prickly pear; NEUTRAL (Allowed Frequently): elderberry (dark blue/purple); AVOID: apple, apricot, date, strawberry.

Spices/Condiments/Sweeteners

Many spices have medicinal properties. Turmeric improves liver function. Garlic improves immune health and is anti-inflammatory, as is cayenne pepper. Parsley contains quercetin, which is anti-inflammatory.

Black pepper can be particularly problematic for allergy sufferers; when the outer covering of the peppercorn is broken, mold can settle on the soft inner core. Many common food additives, such as guar gum and carrageenan, enhance the effects of lectins found in other foods and should be avoided. Use caution when using prepared condiments, as they often contain wheat.

SUPER BENEFICIAL	BENEFICIAL	NEUTRAL: Allowed Frequently	NEUTRAL: Allowed Infrequently	AVOID
Garlic	Carob	Agar	Apple pectin	Aspartame
Parsley	Fenugeek	Allspice	Arrowroot	Caper
Pepper (cayenne)	Ginger	Almond extract	Barley malt	Carrageenan
Turmeric	Horseradish	Anise	Chocolate	Cornstarch
		Basil	Honey	Corn syrup
		Bay leaf	Ketchup	Dextrose
		Bergamot	Maple syrup	Fructose
		Caraway	Molasses	Guarana
		Cardamom	Molasses (blackstrap)	Gums (acacia/ Arabic/ guar)
		Chervil	Rice syrup	Juniper
		Chili powder	Senna	Mace
		Chive	Soy sauce	Maltodextrin
		Cilantro (coriander leaf)	Sucanat	MSG
		Cinnamon		Nutmeg
		Clove		
		Coriander		

SUPER BENEFICIAL	BENEFICIAL	NEUTRAL: Allowed Frequently	NEUTRAL: Allowed Infrequently	AVOID
		Cream of tartar	Sugar (brown/ white)	Pepper (black/ white)
		Cumin		Vinegar (except apple cider)
		Dill		Worcester- shire sauce
		Gelatin, plain		
		Lecithin		
		Licorice root*		
		Marjoram		
		Mayonnaise		
		Mint (all)		
		Mustard (dry)		
		Oregano		
		Paprika		
		Pepper (pepper- corn/red flakes)		
		Rosemary		
		Saffron		
		Sage		
		Savory		
		Sea salt		
		Stevia		
		Tamari (wheat- free)		
		Tamarind		
		Tarragon		
		Thyme		
		Vanilla		

SUPER BENEFICIAL	BENEFICIAL	NEUTRAL: Allowed Frequently	NEUTRAL: Allowed Infrequently	AVOID
		Vegetable glycerine		
		Vinegar (apple cider)		
		Winter-green		
		Yeast (baker's/brewer's)		

Special Variants: *Non-Secretor* BENEFICIAL: basil, bay leaf, licorice root*, oregano, saffron, tarragon, yeast (brewer's); NEUTRAL (Allowed Frequently): carob, MSG, nutmeg, turmeric; AVOID: agar, barley malt, cinnamon, honey, maple syrup, mayonnaise, rice syrup, sage, soy sauce, stevia, sucanat, sugar (brown/white), tamari (wheat-free), vanilla, vinegar (apple cider).

*Do not use if you have high blood pressure.

Herbal Teas

Herbal teas can provide medicinal benefits and are excellent replacements for caffeinated drinks such as coffee, cola, and black tea. SUPER BENEFICIAL herbal teas for Blood Type O help soothe the digestive system.

SUPER BENEFICIAL	BENEFICIAL	NEUTRAL: Allowed Frequently	NEUTRAL: Allowed Infrequently	AVOID
Ginger	Chickweed	Catnip	Senna	Alfalfa
Sarsa-parilla	Dandelion	Chamo-mile		Aloe
Slippery elm	Fenugreek	Dong quai		Burdock
	Hops	Elder		Coltsfoot
	Linden			Corn silk

SUPER BENEFICIAL	BENEFICIAL	NEUTRAL: Allowed Frequently	NEUTRAL: Allowed Infrequently	AVOID
	Mulberry	Ginseng		Echinacea
	Pepper- mint	Hawthorn		Gentian
	Rosehip	Hore- hound		Goldenseal
		Licorice		Red clover
		Mullein		Rhubarb
		Raspberry leaf		Shepherd's purse
		Skullcap		St. John's wort
		Spearmint		Strawberry leaf
		Valerian		Yellow dock
		Vervain		
		White birch		
		White oak bark		
		Yarrow		

Special Variants: None.

Miscellaneous Beverages

Green tea should be part of every Blood Type O's allergy-fighting plan. A compound in green tea, epigallocatechin gallate (EGCG), blocks receptors (IgE and histamine) and is involved in the allergic response. Green tea also contains polyphenols, which enhance gastrointestinal health. Avoid or limit alcohol to an occasional glass of red wine. Eliminate coffee.

SUPER BENEFICIAL	BENEFICIAL	NEUTRAL: Allowed Frequently	NEUTRAL: Allowed Infrequently	AVOID
Tea (green)	Seltzer		Wine (red)	Beer
	Soda (club)			Coffee (reg/ decaf)
				Liquor
				Soda (cola/ diet/misc.)
				Tea, black (reg/decaf)
				Wine (white)

Special Variants: *Non-Secretor* BENEFICIAL: Wine (red).

Supplements

THE BLOOD TYPE O Diet offers abundant quantities of important nutrients, such as protein and iron. It is important to get as many nutrients as possible from fresh foods and use supplements only to fill in the minor deficiencies in your diet. The following supplement protocols are designed for Blood Type O individuals who are suffering from allergies or related conditions.

Note: If you are being treated for a medical condition, consult your doctor before taking any supplements.

Blood Type O
Immune System Health Maintenance

Use this protocol for 4–8 weeks, then discontinue for 2 weeks and restart.

SUPPLEMENT	ACTION	DOSAGE
Larch arabinogalactan	Promotes digestive and intestinal health	1 tblsp, twice daily, in juice or water
Bladderwrack (*Fucus vesiculosus*)	Blocks the activity of complement; lectin blocker	100 mg, twice daily with meals

SUPPLEMENT	ACTION	DOSAGE
Probiotic	Promotes intestinal health	1–2 capsules, twice daily
High-potency vitamin-mineral complex (preferably blood type–specific)	Nutritional support	As directed
Sprouted food complex	Enhances detoxification	1–2 capsules, twice daily

Blood Type O
Specific Allergy Treatment Protocols

Use these protocols for 4–8 weeks, then discontinue for a week and restart. Protocols can be combined.

Anti-Inflammatory/Allergy Relief

SUPPLEMENT	ACTION	DOSAGE
N-acetyl glucosamine (NAG)	Binds inflammatory lectins	250–500 mg, 3–4 times daily, away from food
Frankincense (*Boswellia serrata*)	Has anti-inflammatory effects	500 mg, 1–2 capsules, between meals
Quercetin	Has anti-inflammatory effects; liver protective	500 mg, twice daily, away from meals
SUPPLEMENT	**ACTION**	**DOSAGE**
Stinging nettle leaves (*Urtica dioica*)	Reduces inflammation, skin rashes, eczema	500 mg, 1 capsule, twice daily
Green tea	Blocks pro-inflammatory receptors	1–3 cups daily

Sinus Relief

SUPPLEMENT	ACTION	DOSAGE
MSM (methylsulfo-nylmethane)	Has anti-inflammatory effects	500 mg, 1–2 capsules, twice daily

SUPPLEMENT	ACTION	DOSAGE
Yerba santa (*Eriodictyon californicum*)	Helps eliminate congestion	Tincture: 10–15 drops, twice daily in warm water
Stinging nettle leaves (*Urtica dioica*)	Reduces inflammation, skin rashes, eczema	500 mg, 1 capsule, twice daily

Digestive System Repair

SUPPLEMENT	ACTION	DOSAGE
N-acetyl glucosamine (NAG)	Blocks anti-metabolic lectins in grains and other Blood Type O AVOIDS	300–600 mg, taken with large meals
Quercetin	Has anti-inflammatory effects; liver protective	500 mg, twice daily, away from meals
Bromelain (pineapple enzyme)	Aids digestion	500 mg, 1–3 tablets, 4 times daily between meals, gradually decreasing
Larch arabinogalacfan	Promotes digestive and intestinal health	1 tblsp, twice daily, in juice or water
Bladderwrack (*Fucus vesiculosus*)	Blocks lectin activity	100 mg, 1–2 capsules with meals, 2–5 times daily

Adrenal Support

SUPPLEMENT	ACTION	DOSAGE
Tyrosine	Amino acid, helps balance dopamine/ adrenaline axis	500 mg, twice daily
Ginseng, panax	Great stress/ adrenal tonic	150–200 mg, once or twice daily

The Exercise Component

BLOOD TYPE O benefits tremendously from brisk exercise that taxes the cardiovascular and musculoskeletal systems. Exercise is an immune strengthener, a stress reducer, and a way of reducing total load on the system—a key factor in preventing allergies.

Build a balanced routine of both aerobic and strength-training activities from the following chart. If you are not accustomed to exercising, or you are suffering from a chronic condition, start slowly and do as much as you can, striving to increase your time and endurance as you gain flexibility and strength.

EXERCISE	DURATION	FREQUENCY
Aerobics	40–60 minutes	3–4 x week
Weight training	30–45 minutes	3–4 x week
Running	40–45 minutes	3–4 x week
Calesthenics	30–45 minutes	3 x week
Treadmill	30 minutes	3 x week
Kickboxing	30–45 minutes	3 x week
Cycling	30 minutes	3 x week
Contact sports	60 minutes	2–3 x week
In-line/roller skating	30 minutes	2–3 x week

3 Steps to Effective Exercise

1. Warm up with stretching and flexibility moves before you start your aerobic exercise.
2. To achieve maximum cardiovascular benefits, work toward an elevated heart rate that is about 70 percent of your capacity. Once you reach the elevated rate, continue exercising to maintain that rate for twenty to thirty minutes. To calculate your maximum heart rate and performance level:
   - Subtract your age from 220.
   - Multiply the difference by .70 (or .60 if you are over age sixty). This is the high end of your performance.

- Multiply the remainder by .50. This is the low end of
your performance.
3. Finish each aerobic session with at least a five-minute cool-
down of stretching and relaxation moves.

Getting Started: The First Month

IF YOU ARE NEW to the Blood Type Diet, the following guidelines
will introduce you to the Blood Type O regimen over a period of one
month. Follow these recommendations as closely as possible, using a
notebook to record your personal experiences with the diet. In addition to factors that are measurable in laboratory tests, take the time to
note changes in your energy levels, allergy symptoms, sleep patterns,
digestion, and overall well-being.

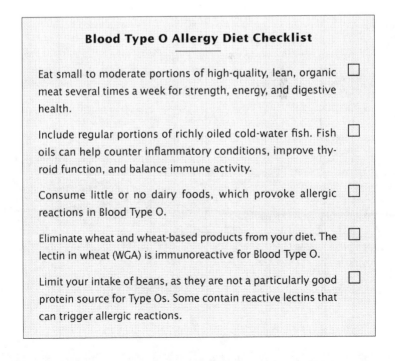

Blood Type O Allergy Diet Checklist

Eat small to moderate portions of high-quality, lean, organic ☐
meat several times a week for strength, energy, and digestive
health.

Include regular portions of richly oiled cold-water fish. Fish ☐
oils can help counter inflammatory conditions, improve thy-
roid function, and balance immune activity.

Consume little or no dairy foods, which provoke allergic ☐
reactions in Blood Type O.

Eliminate wheat and wheat-based products from your diet. The ☐
lectin in wheat (WGA) is immunoreactive for Blood Type O.

Limit your intake of beans, as they are not a particularly good ☐
protein source for Type Os. Some contain reactive lectins that
can trigger allergic reactions.

Eat lots of BENEFICIAL fruits and vegetables.   ☐

Avoid coffee, but drink green tea every day. It contains com-   ☐
pounds that block IgE and histamine.

Avoid foods that are Type O allergy red flags, especially wheat,   ☐
corn, kidney beans, navy beans, lentils, peanuts, potatoes,
and cauliflower.

Week 1

Blood Type Diet and Supplements

- Eliminate your most harmful AVOID foods—wheat and dairy. These foods
  are the primary triggers for inflammatory conditions.

- Include your most important BENEFICIAL foods on a regular schedule
  throughout the week. For example, have lean red meat 5 times, and omega-
  3-rich fish 3 to 4 times, with lots of BENEFICIAL vegetables and fruit.

- Incorporate at least 1 SUPER BENEFICIAL food into your daily diet. For example, eat slices of fresh pineapple or a seaweed salad.

- If you're a coffee drinker, begin to wean yourself by cutting your daily consumption in half. Substitute green tea or 1 of the SUPER BENEFICIAL herbal
  teas, such as ginger or sarsaparilla.

Exercise Regimen

- Plan to exercise at least 4 days this week, for 45 minutes each day.

  2 days: aerobic activity

  2 days: weights

- If you feel exhausted by the symptoms of allergies, start slowly and gradually increase the duration and intensity of your activity. The important factor is consistency. Just do it—as much as you're able. If allergy to grasses
  and weeds prevents outdoor activities, such as walking and running, join an
  aerobics class or walk around the track at your local gym.

- Use your journal to detail the time, activity, distance, and amount of weight
  lifted. Note the number of repetitions for each exercise.

■ **WEEK 1 SUCCESS STRATEGY** ■
Neti Pots for Clear and Healthy Sinuses

Neti is the Ayurvedic and yoga practice of cleansing the nasal passages. Using a specially designed neti pot is a safe and effective way to perform this cleansing routine. A neti pot is a small pot with a spout that fits into the nostril and seals it.

- Fill the pot with lukewarm water and dissolve a teaspoon of ordinary salt (not sea salt) in the water.
- Stand over a sink, placing the spout against one nostril, so that it fits tightly. Lean forward, breathe relaxed through the mouth, and turn the head to one side. The water will flow by itself, in through one nostril and out of the other.
- When half of the water has run through one nostril, gently blow out any remaining water and mucus. Then repeat this process in the other nostril.
- After performing the process on both nostrils, bend forward and let your head hang loosely down, so that the remaining water can run out of the nose. Close one nostril with the index finger and turn the head alternating from side to side. Blow gently through one nostril at a time until the nose is dry.

There are a number of Internet sites that sell neti pots. You can also purchase them at yoga centers and at some health-food stores.

Week 2

Blood Type Diet and Supplements

- Begin to eliminate the next level of AVOID foods—corn, potatoes, beans, and legumes.
- Eat at least 2 BENEFICIAL animal proteins every day, choosing from the meat, poultry, and seafood lists.
- Initially, it is best to avoid foods listed as NEUTRAL: Allowed Infrequently.
- Continue to incorporate SUPER BENEFICIAL foods into your daily diet.

- If you're a coffee drinker, continue to cut your coffee intake. Replace it with green tea. Two to 3 cups of green tea each day can help counter sinus problems.
- Manage your mealtimes to aid proper digestion. Avoid eating on the run. Make your meals relaxing, sit-down affairs. Eat slowly and chew thoroughly to encourage digestive secretions.

Exercise Regimen

- Continue to exercise at least 4 days this week, for 45 minutes each day.

  2 days: aerobic activity

  2 days: weights

- If your work is sedentary, get in the habit of taking a couple of "movement" breaks during the day. Walk around the block, or take the stairs instead of the elevator.

■ WEEK 2 SUCCESS STRATEGY ■
Nip Allergy Symptoms in the Bud

In addition to practicing lectin-avoidance with the Type O Diet, take these measures at the first sign of allergies:

- Take a teaspoon of rosehip concentrate and continue every thirty minutes as needed.
- Drink one to two cups of stinging nettle leaf tea daily while symptoms continue.

Week 3

Blood Type Diet and Supplements

- When you plan your meals for week 3, choose BENEFICIAL or SUPER BENEFI-CIAL foods to replace NEUTRAL foods whenever possible. For example, choose lean, organic beef or buffalo over chicken, or blueberries over an apple.
- Eliminate all remaining AVOID foods.
- Liberally incorporate SUPER BENEFICIAL foods into your daily diet.
- Completely wean yourself from coffee, substituting green tea or herbal tea.

Exercise Regimen

- Continue to exercise at least 4 days this week, for 45 minutes each day.

  2 days: aerobic activity

  2 days: weights

■ WEEK 3 SUCCESS STRATEGY ■
Allergy-Proof Your Home

- Always wash bedding in hot water (at least 130° F) to kill dust mites. Cold water won't do the job. Launder bedding at least every seven to ten days.

- Use synthetic or foam rubber mattress pads and pillows, and plastic mattress covers if you are allergic. Do not use fuzzy wool blankets, feather or wool-stuffed comforters, or feather pillows.

- Clean rooms and closets well; dust and vacuum often to remove surface dust. Vacuuming and other cleaning may not remove all animal dander, dust mite material, and other biological pollutants. Some particles are so small they can pass through vacuum bags and remain in the air. If you are allergic to dust, wear a mask when vacuuming or dusting.

- Clean mold surfaces, such as showers and kitchen counters.

- Remove mold from walls, ceilings, floors, and paneling. Do not simply cover mold with paint, stain, varnish, or a moisture-proof sealer, as it may resurface.

- Throw out wicker furniture, straw baskets, and the like that have been water damaged or contain mold. These cannot be recovered.

- Discard any water-damaged furnishings such as carpets, drapes, stuffed toys, upholstered furniture, and ceiling tiles, unless they can be recovered by steam cleaning or hot water washing and thorough drying.

- Remove and replace wet insulation to prevent conditions where biological pollutants can grow.

- Household chemicals may be harmful if swallowed or inhaled. Avoid contact with skin, eyes, mucous membranes, and clothing.

Week 4

Blood Type Diet and Supplements

- Continue at the week 3 level, focusing on BENEFICIAL and SUPER BENEFICIAL foods.
- Evaluate the first 4 weeks and make adjustments.

Exercise Regimen

- Continue at the week 3 level.
- Review your progress, noting in your journal improvements in strength, flexibility, and overall energy. Determine which exercise regimen has worked for you, including time of day, setting, and activity level.

■ **WEEK 4 SUCCESS STRATEGY** ■
Travel in Comfort

The American Academy of Allergy, Asthma and Immunology (AAAAI) publishes a report from the National Allergy Bureau (1-800-POLLEN), "Pollen and Spores around the World," which is packed with information about seasonal patterns in the United States and around the world. This information can help you plan vacations and business trips for times when pollen and mold counts are the lowest.

A Final Word

IN SUMMARY, the secret to fighting allergies with the Blood Type O Diet involves:

1. Maximizing overall health by adhering to a diet that is animal protein–based.
2. Minimizing the consumption of allergy-producing lectins, most abundant in grains such as wheat.
3. Increasing strength, flexibility, and circulatory efficiency by adopting a vigorous exercise program.
4. Using supplements to block the effects of pro-inflammatory lectins, provide antioxidant support, and balance immune activity.

Blood Type

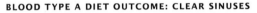

BLOOD TYPE A DIET OUTCOME: CLEAR SINUSES

"I was on antibiotics and decongestants regularly for years for sinus infections. I noticed a change on the fifth day of the diet and have taken no decongestants or antibiotics since. I had been diagnosed with fibrocystic breast disease, and at about one month on the diet, most of the cysts/lumps were gone."

BLOOD TYPE A DIET OUTCOME: DECONGESTANTS BEGONE

"I have been to every doctor in the state, it seems, for allergies and sinus infections. After years of antibiotics, decongestants, and pain relievers, I was fed up. Since I started the Blood Type Diet, I haven't taken even one decongestant or pain reliever. I am amazed!"

BLOOD TYPE A DIET OUTCOME: NEW IMMUNE STRENGTH

"Following the Blood Type A Diet has improved my nose, ears, throat, et al. My sensitivity to allergens (cats, dust, mold) has diminished. I feel that my body has also been immunologically improved. Making changes was not exceedingly difficult, as I was a fish-eating vegetarian already. Cutting out tomatoes, wheat, and dairy has been the most difficult."

Self-reported outcomes from the Blood Type Diet Web site (www.dadamo.com)

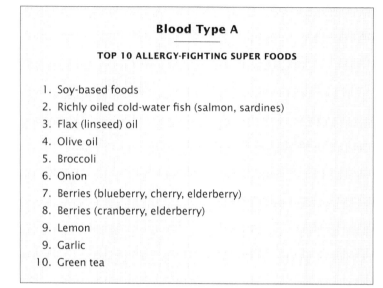

Blood Type A

TOP 10 ALLERGY-FIGHTING SUPER FOODS

1. Soy-based foods
2. Richly oiled cold-water fish (salmon, sardines)
3. Flax (linseed) oil
4. Olive oil
5. Broccoli
6. Onion
7. Berries (blueberry, cherry, elderberry)
8. Berries (cranberry, elderberry)
9. Lemon
9. Garlic
10. Green tea

Blood Type A: The Foods

THE BLOOD TYPE A Allergy Diet is specifically adapted for the prevention and management of allergies. A new category, **Super Beneficial,** highlights powerful disease-fighting foods for Blood Type A. The **Neutral** category has also been adjusted to de-emphasize foods that are less advantageous for you. Foods designated **Neutral: Allowed Infrequently** should be minimized or avoided entirely.

Your secretor status can influence your ability to fully digest and metabolize certain foods, so various adjustments in the values are made for non-secretors. If you do not know your secretor type, the odds are that you can safely use the "secretor" values, since the majority of the population (approximately 80 percent) are secretors. However, I urge you to get tested, since the variations are important for non-secretors who want to maximize the effectiveness of the Blood Type Diet. To find out how to get tested, visit our Web site (www.dadamo.com).

The food charts are divided into three sections. The top of the chart suggests the average portion size and quantity per week or day, according to secretor status. These recommendations do *not* apply to the category **Neutral: Allowed Infrequently;** those foods should be eaten rarely, if at all. The charts also indicate differences in frequency for some foods based on ethnic heritage. It has been my experience that this factor has an impact upon the individual's ability to fully digest certain foods. For the purposes of blood type food choices, persons of Hispanic heritage should follow the guidelines for Caucasians, and American Native peoples should follow the guidelines for Asians.

The middle section of the chart gives the food values. The bottom section lists variants based on secretor status.

For your convenience, we have included a number of product names (Ezekiel 4:9 bread, Worcestershire sauce, etc.). However, keep in mind that commercial formulations vary among brands and regions. Even though a product may be listed as acceptable for you, always check its ingredients. Some products may contain **Avoid** ingredients for your blood type. Of course, you may choose to make your own version of commercial products, such as bread and mayonnaise, using ingredients that suit your blood type. There are hundreds of delicious recipes for every blood type available on our Web site (www. dadamo.com) and in the book *Cook Right 4 Your Type: The Practical Kitchen Companion to* Eat Right 4 Your Type.

Meat/Poultry

Blood Type A lacks some of the enzymes and stomach acids needed to effectively digest animal protein. When you overconsume meat, the undigested by-products can create a toxic environment. Allergies can be triggered or enhanced by the ensuing gastrointestinal conditions. For this reason you should derive most of your protein from non-meat sources. Non-secretors have a small advantage over secretors in the ability to digest animal protein but should still derive most of their protein from foods other than meat. Choose only the best quality (preferably free-range), chemical-, antibiotic-, and pesticide-free low-fat meats and poultry.

BLOOD TYPE A: MEAT/POULTRY

Portion: 4–6 oz (men); 2–5 oz (women and children)

	African	Caucasian	Asian
Secretor	0–2	0–3	0–3
Non-Secretor	2–5	2–4	2–3
		Times per week	

SUPER BENEFICIAL	BENEFICIAL	NEUTRAL: Allowed Frequently	NEUTRAL: Allowed Infrequently	AVOID
		Chicken		All commercially processed meats
		Cornish hen		Bacon/ham/pork
		Grouse		Beef
		Guinea hen		Buffalo
		Ostrich		Duck
		Squab		Goat
		Turkey		Goose
				Heart (beef)
				Horse
				Lamb
				Liver (calf)
				Mutton
				Partridge
				Pheasant
				Quail
				Rabbit
				Squirrel
				Sweetbreads
				Turtle

SUPER BENEFICIAL	BENEFICIAL	NEUTRAL: Allowed Frequently	NEUTRAL: Allowed Infrequently	AVOID
				Veal
				Venison

Special Variants: *Non-Secretor* BENEFICIAL: turkey; NEUTRAL (Allowed Frequently): duck, goat, goose, lamb, mutton, partridge, pheasant, quail, rabbit, turtle.

Fish/Seafood

Fish and seafood represent a nutritious source of protein for Blood Type A. SUPER BENEFICIAL are the richly oiled cold-water fish, such as cod, mackerel, salmon, sardines, and trout. These are rich in omega-3 fatty acids, such as docosahexaenoic acid (DHA) and eicosapentaenoic acid (EPA), which can help to balance immune function and reduce inflammation. Avoid most shellfish, as they can trigger allergic reactions.

BLOOD TYPE A: FISH/SEAFOOD			
Portion: 4–6 oz (men); 2–5 oz (women and children)			
	African	Caucasian	Asian
Secretor	1–3	1–3	1–3
Non-Secretor	2–5	2–5	2–4
	Times per week		

SUPER BENEFICIAL	BENEFICIAL	NEUTRAL: Allowed Frequently	NEUTRAL: Allowed Infrequently	AVOID
Cod	Carp	Abalone		Anchovy
Mackerel	Monkfish	Bass (sea)		Barracuda
Salmon	Perch (silver/ yellow)	Bullhead		Bass (bluegill/ striped)
Sardine		Butterfish		
		Chub		

SUPER BENEFICIAL	BENEFICIAL	NEUTRAL: Allowed Frequently	NEUTRAL: Allowed Infrequently	AVOID
Trout (rainbow)	Pickerel	Croaker		Beluga
	Pollock	Cusk		Bluefish
	Red snapper	Drum		Catfish
	Snail (*Helix pomatia/* escargot)	Halfmoon fish		Caviar (sturgeon)
	Trout (sea)	Mahi-mahi		Clam
	Whitefish	Mullet		Conch
	Whiting	Muskellunge		Crab
		Orange roughy		Crayfish
		Parrot fish		Eel
		Perch (white)		Flounder
		Pike		Frog
		Pompano		Gray sole
		Porgy		Grouper
		Rosefish		Haddock
		Sailfish		Hake
		Salmon roe		Halibut
		Scrod		Harvest fish
		Shark		Herring (fresh/ pickled/ smoked)
		Smelt		Lobster
		Sturgeon		Mussel
		Sucker		Octopus
		Sunfish		Opaleye
		Swordfish		Oyster
		Tilapia		Salmon (smoked)
		Trout (brook)		Scallop
		Tuna		Scup
		Weakfish		Shad
				Shrimp

SUPER BENEFICIAL	BENEFICIAL	NEUTRAL: Allowed Frequently	NEUTRAL: Allowed Infrequently	AVOID
		Yellowtail		Sole
				Squid (calamari)
				Tilefish

Special Variants: *Non-Secretor* BENEFICIAL: chub, cusk, drum, halfmoon fish, harvest fish, mullet, muskellunge, perch (white), pompano, rosefish, sailfish, sucker, swordfish, trout (brook); NEUTRAL (Allowed Frequently): anchovy, bass (bluegill), beluga, bluefish, caviar (sturgeon), flounder, frog, gray sole, grouper, haddock, hake, halibut, herring (fresh), mussel, octopus, opaleye, scallop, scup, shad, tilefish.

Dairy/Eggs

Dairy foods should mostly be avoided by Blood Type A, especially those with allergies or sinus problems related to excess mucus production. Eggs can be consumed in moderation, unless they produce allergic reactions. Do your best to find eggs and dairy products that are both hormone-free and organic.

BLOOD TYPE A: EGGS			
Portion: 1 egg			
	African	Caucasian	Asian
Secretor	1–3	1–3	1–3
Non-Secretor	2–3	2–5	2–4
			Times per week

BLOOD TYPE A: MILK AND YOGURT			
Portion: 4–6 oz (men); 2–5 oz (women and children)			
	African	Caucasian	Asian
Secretor	0–1	1–3	0–3
Non-Secretor	0–1	1–2	0–2
			Times per week

BLOOD TYPE A: CHEESE

Portion: 4–6 oz (men); 2–5 oz (women and children)

	African	Caucasian	Asian
Secretor	0–2	1–3	0–2
Non-Secretor	0	0–1	0–1
		Times per week	

SUPER BENEFICIAL	BENEFICIAL	NEUTRAL: Allowed Frequently	NEUTRAL: Allowed Infrequently	AVOID
		Egg (chicken/ duck/ goose/ quail) Farmer cheese Ghee (clarified butter) Kefir Mozzarella Paneer Ricotta Yogurt	Feta Goat cheese Milk (goat) Sour cream	American cheese Blue cheese Brie Butter Buttermilk Camembert Casein Cheddar Colby Cottage cheese Cream cheese Edam Emmenthal Gouda Gruyère Half-and- half Ice cream Jarlsberg Milk (cow) Monterey Jack Muenster

SUPER BENEFICIAL	BENEFICIAL	NEUTRAL: Allowed Frequently	NEUTRAL: Allowed Infrequently	AVOID
				Neufchâtel
				Parmesan
				Provolone
				Sherbet
				Swiss cheese
				Whey

Special Variants: *Non-Secretor* NEUTRAL (Allowed Frequently): cottage cheese, whey; AVOID: milk (goat), sour cream.

Oils

Olive oil, a monounsaturated fat, is SUPER BENEFICIAL for Blood Type A. Constituents in olive oil, such as flavonoids, squalenes, and polyphenols, act as powerful antioxidants. It should be used as a primary cooking oil. Also SUPER BENEFICIAL is flax (linseed) oil, which is high in alpha-linolenic acid (ALA) and has anti-inflammatory properties.

Be aware that some oils are high in omega-6 fatty acids, which can stimulate the inflammatory response. These include corn, cottonseed, and peanut oils.

BLOOD TYPE A: OILS			
Portion: 1 tblsp			
	African	Caucasian	Asian
Secretor	5–8	5–8	5–8
Non-Secretor	3–7	3–7	3–6
	Times per week		

SUPER BENEFICIAL	BENEFICIAL	NEUTRAL: Allowed Frequently	NEUTRAL: Allowed Infrequently	AVOID
Flax (linseed) Olive	Black currant seed Walnut	Almond Borage seed Cod liver Evening primrose Safflower Sesame Soy Sunflower Wheat germ	Canola	Castor Coconut Corn Cottonseed Peanut

Special Variants: *Non-Secretor* BENEFICIAL: cod liver, sesame; NEUTRAL (Allowed Frequently): peanut; AVOID: safflower.

Nuts/Seeds

Nuts and seeds can serve as an important secondary source of protein for Blood Type A. Laboratory research has identified at least five natural phytochemicals in nuts that regulate the immune system and act as antioxidants. SUPER BENEFICIAL for Blood Type A are flax seeds and walnuts, which are high in omega-3 fatty acids.

BLOOD TYPE A: NUTS/SEEDS			
Portion: Whole (handful); Nut Butters (2 tblsp)			
	African	Caucasian	Asian
Secretor	4–7	4–7	4–7
Non-Secretor	5–7	5–7	5–7
	Times per week		

SUPER BENEFICIAL	BENEFICIAL	NEUTRAL: Allowed Frequently	NEUTRAL: Allowed Infrequently	AVOID
Flax	Peanut	Almond	Safflower seed	Brazil nut
Walnut (black/ English)	Peanut butter	Almond butter	Sesame butter (tahini)	Cashew
	Pumpkin seed	Almond cheese	Sesame seed	Pistachio
		Almond milk		
		Beechnut		
		Butternut		
		Chestnut		
		Filbert (hazel- nut)		
		Hickory nut		
		Litchi		
		Macadamia nut		
		Pecan		
		Pignolia (pine nut)		
		Poppy seed		
		Sunflower butter		
		Sunflower seed		

Special Variants: *Non-Secretor* AVOID: safflower seed, sunflower butter, sunflower seed.

Beans/Legumes

Blood Type A thrives on vegetable proteins found in many beans and legumes, although a few beans contain immunoreactive proteins and should be avoided. SUPER BENEFICIAL beans and legumes for Blood Type A include soy beans and their by-products. They are a good source of essential amino acids, and they contain isoflavones that can inhibit inflammation-inducing selectins from being overexpressed on the blood vessels.

BLOOD TYPE A: BEANS/LEGUMES			
Portion: 1 cup (cooked)			
	African	Caucasian	Asian
Secretor	5–7	5–7	5–7
Non-Secretor	3–5	3–5	3–5
		Times per week	

SUPER BENEFICIAL	BENEFICIAL	NEUTRAL: Allowed Frequently	NEUTRAL: Allowed Infrequently	AVOID
Soy bean	Adzuki bean	Cannellini bean		Copper bean
Soy cheese	Bean (green/ snap/ string)	Jicama bean		Garbanzo (chickpea)
Soy milk		Mung bean/ sprouts		Kidney bean
Soy, miso	Black bean			Lima bean
Soy, tempeh	Black-eyed pea	Northern bean		Navy bean
Soy, tofu	Fava (broad) bean	Pea (green/ pod/ snow)		Tamarind bean
	Lentil (all)			
	Pinto bean	White bean		

Special Variants: *Non-Secretor* NEUTRAL (Allowed Frequently): adzuki bean, bean (green/snap/string), black bean, black-eyed pea, copper bean, fava (broad) bean, kidney bean, navy bean, soy bean and products.

Grains/Starches

Blood Type A benefits from a moderate consumption of grains. If you have allergies, you should limit or avoid wheat and corn products. This is especially important for non-secretors. The agglutinin in whole wheat can aggravate inflammatory conditions and derail the proper response of the immune system. This lectin can sometimes be milled out of the grain or destroyed by sprouting.

BLOOD TYPE A: GRAINS/STARCHES

Portion: ½ cup dry (grains or pastas); 1 muffin; 2 slices of bread

	African	Caucasian	Asian
Secretor	7–10	7–9	7–10
Non-Secretor	5–7	5–7	5–7
	Times per week		

SUPER BENEFICIAL	BENEFICIAL	NEUTRAL: Allowed Frequently	NEUTRAL: Allowed Infrequently	AVOID
	Amaranth	Barley	Cornmeal	Telf
	Buckwheat	Kamut	Couscous	Wheat bran
	Essene bread (manna)	Quinoa	Grits	Wheat germ
	Ezekiel 4:9 bread	Rice (wild)	Millet	
	Oat bran	Rice cake	Popcorn	
	Oat flour	Rice flour/ products	Tapioca	
	Oatmeal	Rice milk	Wheat (whole)	
	Rice (whole)	Rye flour/ products	Wheat (refined/ unbleached)	
	Rice bran	Sorghum	Wheat (semolina)	
	Rye (whole)	Spelt (whole)	Wheat (white flour)	
		Spelt flour/ products		

SUPER BENEFICIAL	BENEFICIAL	NEUTRAL: Allowed Frequently	NEUTRAL: Allowed Infrequently	AVOID
	Soba noodles (100% buck- wheat) Soy flour/ products		100% sprouted grain products (except Essene, Ezekiel)	

Special Variants: *Non-Secretor* NEUTRAL (Allowed Frequently): buckwheat, Ezekiel 4:9 bread, oat (all), soba noodles (100% buckwheat), soy flour/products, teff; AVOID: cornmeal, couscous, grits, popcorn, wheat (all).

Vegetables

Vegetables provide a rich source of antioxidants and fiber and are crucial to intestinal health. Onions are SUPER BENEFICIAL for Type A. They contain significant amounts of the antioxidant quercetin.

Tomatoes contain a lectin that reacts with the saliva and digestive juices of Blood Type A secretors, although it does not appear to react with non-secretors. Yams are typically high in the amino acid phenylalanine, which inactivates intestinal alkaline phosphatase (already quite low in Blood Type A) and should be avoided.

An item's value also applies to its juices, unless otherwise noted.

BLOOD TYPE A: VEGETABLES

Portion: 1 cup, prepared (cooked or raw)

	African	Caucasian	Asian
Secretor Super/Beneficials	Unlimited	Unlimited	Unlimited
Secretor Neutrals	2–5	2–5	2–5
Non-Secretor Super/Beneficials	Unlimited	Unlimited	Unlimited
Non-Secretor Neutrals	2–3	2–3	2–3
		Times per day	

SUPER BENEFICIAL	BENEFICIAL	NEUTRAL: Allowed Frequently	NEUTRAL: Allowed Infrequently	AVOID
Broccoli	Alfalfa	Arugula	Corn	Cabbage
Celery	sprouts	Asparagus	Olive	Eggplant
Kale	Aloe	Asparagus	(green)	Mushroom
Onion (all)	Artichoke	pea	Pickle (in	(shiitake)
Spinach	Beet	Bamboo	brine)	Olive
Swiss	Beet	shoot	Squash	(black/
chard	greens	Beet	(all)	Greek/
	Carrot	Bok choy		Spanish)
	Chicory	Brussels		Peppers (all)
	Collards	sprouts		Pickle (in
	Dandelion	Cabbage		vinegar)
	Escarole	(juice)*		Potato
	Horse-	Cauliflower		Potato
	radish	Celeriac		(sweet)
	Kohlrabi	Cucumber		Rhubarb
	Leek	Daikon		Tomato
	Lettuce	radish		Yam
	(Romaine)	Endive		Yucca
	Mushroom	Fennel		
	(maitake/	Fiddlehead		
	silver	fern		
	dollar)	Lettuce		
	Okra	(except		
	Parsnip	Romaine)		
	Pumpkin	Mung		
	Rappini	bean/		
	(broccoli	sprouts		
	rabe)	Mushroom		
	Turnip	(abalone/		
		enoki/		
		oyster/		
		porto-		
		bello/		
		straw/		
		tree ear)		

SUPER BENEFICIAL	BENEFICIAL	NEUTRAL: Allowed Frequently	NEUTRAL: Allowed Infrequently	AVOID
		Mustard greens		
		Oyster plant		
		Poi		
		Radicchio		
		Radish/ sprouts		
		Rutabaga		
		Scallion		
		Seaweeds		
		Shallot		
		Taro		
		Water chestnut		
		Watercress		
		Zucchini		

Special Variants: *Non-Secretor* NEUTRAL (Allowed Frequently): alfalfa sprouts, aloe, carrot, celery, eggplant, garlic, horseradish, lettuce (Romaine), mushroom (maitake/shiitake), peppers (all), potato (sweet), rappini (broccoli rabe), taro, tomato; AVOID: agar, cabbage (juice), mushroom (silver dollar), pickle (in brine).

*To obtain the benefits of cabbage juice, it must be consumed within one minute of juicing.

Fruits and Fruit Juices

Fruits are rich in antioxidants, especially blueberries, elderberries, cherries, and blackberries. Pineapple contains useful digestive enzymes. Lemon is an effective mucus reducer. Plums and prunes are high in the phytonutrients neochlorogenic and chlorogenic acids. These substances are classified as phenols, and their function as antioxidants has been well-documented. Several fruits, such as bananas and oranges, contain Blood Type A–reactive lectins, and these should be avoided.

An item's value also applies to its juice, unless otherwise noted.

BLOOD TYPE A: FRUITS AND FRUIT JUICES

Portion: 1 cup

	African	Caucasian	Asian
Secretor	2–4	3–4	3–4
Non-Secretor	2–3	2–3	2–3
	Times per day		

SUPER BENEFICIAL	BENEFICIAL	NEUTRAL: Allowed Frequently	NEUTRAL: Allowed Infrequently	AVOID
Blackberry	Apricot	Apple	Currant	Banana
Blueberry	Boysen-	Asian pear	Date	Bitter melon
Cherry	berry	Avocado	Grape (all)	Coconut
Elderberry	Cranberry	Breadfruit	Pome-	Honeydew
(dark	Fig (fresh/	Canang	granate	Mango
blue/	dried)	melon	Quince	Orange
purple)	Grapefruit	Canta-	Raisin	Papaya
Lemon	Lime	loupe	Star fruit	Plantain
Pineapple		Casaba	(caram-	Tangerine
Plum		melon	bola)	
Prune		Christmas	Strawberry	
		melon		
		Cranberry		
		(juice)		
		Crenshaw		
		melon		
		Dewberry		
		Goose-		
		berry		
		Guava		
		Kiwi		
		Kumquat		
		Logan-		
		berry		
		Mulberry		
		Musk-		
		melon		

SUPER BENEFICIAL	BENEFICIAL	NEUTRAL: Allowed Frequently	NEUTRAL: Allowed Infrequently	AVOID
		Nectarine		
		Peach		
		Pear		
		Persian melon		
		Persimmon		
		Prickly pear		
		Raspberry		
		Sago palm		
		Spanish melon		
		Water- melon		
		Young- berry		

Special Variants: *Non-Secretor* BENEFICIAL: cranberry (juice), elderberry (dark blue/purple), watermelon; NEUTRAL (Allowed Frequently): banana, coconut, lime, mango, plantain, tangerine; AVOID: cantaloupe, casaba melon.

Spices/Condiments/Sweeteners

Many spices have medicinal properties. Turmeric improves liver function. Garlic improves immune health and is anti-inflammatory. Ginger is anti-inflammatory and aids digestive health. Parsley contains quercetin, which is anti-inflammatory. Many common food additives, such as guar gum and carrageenan, enhance the effects of lectins found in other foods and should be avoided.

SUPER BENEFICIAL	BENEFICIAL	NEUTRAL: Allowed Frequently	NEUTRAL: Allowed Infrequently	AVOID
Garlic	Barley malt	Agar	Brown rice syrup	Aspartame
Ginger	Coriander seeds	Allspice	Chocoate	Caper
Parsley	Fenugreek	Almond extract	Cornstarch	Carrageenan
Turmeric	Horse-radish	Anise	Corn syrup	Chili powder
	Molasses (black-strap)	Apple pectin	Dextrose	Gelatin (except veg-sourced)
	Mustard (dry)	Arrowroot	Fructose	
	Soy sauce	Basil	Guarana	Gums (acacia/ Arabic/ guar)
	Tamari (wheat-free)	Bay leaf	Honey	
		Bergamot	Malto-dextrin	Juniper
		Caraway	Maple syrup	Ketchup
		Cardamon	Rice syrup	Mayonnaise
		Carob	Senna	MSG
		Chervil	Sugar (brown/ white)	Pepper (black/ white)
		Chive		
		Cilantro (corian-der leaf)		Pepper (cayenne)
		Cinnamon		Pepper (pepper-corn/ red flakes)
		Clove		
		Cream of tartar		Pickles/ relish
		Cumin		Sucanat
		Dill		Vinegar (all)
		Invert sugar		Wintergreen
		Licorice root*		Worcester-shire sauce
		Mace		
		Marjoram		
		Mint (all)		
		Molasses		

SUPER BENEFICIAL	BENEFICIAL	NEUTRAL: Allowed Frequently	NEUTRAL: Allowed Infrequently	AVOID
		Nutmeg		
		Oregano		
		Paprika		
		Rosemary		
		Saffron		
		Sage		
		Savory		
		Sea salt		
		Seaweeds		
		Stevia		
		Tamarind		
		Tarragon		
		Thyme		
		Vanilla		
		Vegetable glycerine		
		Yeast (baker's/ brewer's)		

Special Variants: *Non-Secretor* BENEFICIAL: cilantro (coriander leaf), yeast (brewer's); NEUTRAL (Allowed Frequently): barley malt, chili powder, molasses, parsley, rice syrup, soy sauce, tamari (wheat-free), turmeric, wintergreen; AVOID: agar, cornstarch, corn syrup, dextrose, invert sugar, maltodextrin, senna.

*Do not use if you have high blood pressure.

Herbal Teas

Many herbal teas are anti-inflammatory. These include ginger, fenugreek, and holy basil. Echinacea and rosehip tea can support immune health.

SUPER BENEFICIAL	BENEFICIAL	NEUTRAL: Allowed Frequently	NEUTRAL: Allowed Infrequently	AVOID
Chamomile	Alfalfa	Chickweed	Hops	Catnip
Dandelion	Aloe	Coltsfoot	Senna	Cayenne
Echinacea	Burdock	Dong quai		Corn silk
Fenugreek	Gentian	Elderberry		Red clover
Ginger	Ginkgo biloba	Goldenseal		Rhubarb
Holy basil	Ginseng	Horehound		Yellow dock
Rosehip	Hawthorn	Licorice root*		
	Milk thistle	Linden		
	Parsley	Mulberry		
	Slippery elm	Mullein		
	St. John's wort	Peppermint		
	Stone root	Raspberry leaf		
	Valerian	Sage		
		Sarsaparilla		
		Shepherd's purse		
		Skullcap		
		Spearmint		
		Strawberry leaf		
		Thyme		
		White birch		
		White oak bark		
		Yarrow		

Special Variants: *Non-Secretor* AVOID: senna.

*Avoid if you have high blood pressure.

Miscellaneous Beverages

Green tea is a SUPER BENEFICIAL beverage for Blood Type A because of its antioxidant properties. It also contains epigallocatechin gallate (EGCG), which blocks receptors involved in the allergic response (IgE and histamine). Red wine contains gallic acid, trans-resveratrol, quercetin, and rutin—four phenolic compounds with potent antioxidant effects. Blood Type A individuals who are not caffeine sensitive might consider having one cup of coffee daily; it contains many enzymes, also found in soy, that can help your immune system function more effectively.

SUPER BENEFICIAL	BENEFICIAL	NEUTRAL: Allowed Frequently	NEUTRAL: Allowed Infrequently	AVOID
Tea (green)	Coffee (reg)	Coffee (decaf)		Beer
	Wine (red)	Wine (white)		Liquor
				Seltzer
				Soda (club)
				Soda (cola/diet/ misc.)
				Tea, black (reg/decaf)

Special Variants: *Non-Secretor* BENEFICIAL: wine (white); NEUTRAL (Allowed Frequently): beer, seltzer, soda (club), tea, black (reg/decaf).

Supplements

THE BLOOD TYPE A Diet offers abundant quantities of important nutrients, such as protein and iron. It is important to get as many nutrients as possible from fresh foods and use supplements only to fill in the minor deficiencies in your diet. The following supplement protocols are designed for Blood Type A individuals who are suffering from allergies or related conditions.

Note: If you are being treated for a medical condition, consult your doctor before taking any supplements.

Blood Type A
Immune System Health Maintenance

Use this protocol for 4–8 weeks, then discontinue for 2 weeks and restart.

SUPPLEMENT	ACTION	DOSAGE
Larch arabinogalactan	Promotes digestive and intestinal health	1 tblsp, twice daily, in juice or water
Probiotic	Promotes intestinal health	1–2 capsules, twice daily
High-potency vitamin-mineral complex (preferably blood type–specific)	Nutritional support	As directed
Sprouted food complex	Enhances detoxification	1–2 capsules, twice daily
Vitamin C	Acts as an antioxidant	250 mg daily, from rosehips or acerola cherry

Blood Type A
Specific Allergy Treatment Protocols

Use these protocols for 4–8 weeks, then discontinue for a week and restart. Protocols can be combined.

Anti-Inflammatory/Allergy Relief

SUPPLEMENT	ACTION	DOSAGE
Hawthorn root (*Crataegus spp.*)	Has anti-inflammatory effects, anti-allergy effects in Type A	Solid extract: ¼ tsp, twice daily Tincture: 20 drops, twice daily
Quercetin	Has anti-inflammatory effects; liver protective	500 mg, twice daily, away from meals
Stinging nettle leaves (*Urtica dioica*)	Reduces inflammation, skin rashes, eczema	500 mg, 1 capsule, twice daily
Green tea	Blocks pro-inflammatory receptors	1–3 cups daily

Sinus Relief

SUPPLEMENT	ACTION	DOSAGE
Stone root (*Collinsonia canadensis*)	Supports sinus health	200 mg, 1–2 capsules, twice daily
Quercetin	Has anti-inflammatory effects; liver protective	500 mg, twice daily, away from meals
Stinging nettle leaves (*Urtica dioica*)	Reduces inflammation, skin rashes, eczema	500 mg, 1 capsule, twice daily

Digestive System Repair

SUPPLEMENT	ACTION	DOSAGE
Quercetin	Has anti-inflammatory effects; liver protective	500 mg, twice daily, away from meals

SUPPLEMENT	ACTION	DOSAGE
Bromelain (pineapple enzyme)	Aids digestion	500 mg, 1–3 tablets, 4 times daily between meals, gradually decreasing
Larch arabinogalactan	Promotes digestive and intestinal health	1 tblsp, twice daily, in juice or water
Adrenal Support		
SUPPLEMENT	ACTION	DOSAGE
Spreading hogweed (*Boerhaavia diffusa*)	Acts as a stress modifier and a liver protector; lowers cortisol	50–150 mg, twice daily
Holy basil (*Ocimum sanctum*) leaf extract	Lowers cortisol	50 mg, twice daily
Pantothenic acid (vitamin B_5)	Stress/adrenal support	50–100 mg, twice daily

The Exercise Component

FOR BLOOD TYPE A, overall fitness, clear breathing, and immune health depend on engaging in regular exercises, with an emphasis on calming exercises such as Hatha yoga and T'ai Chi, as well as light aerobic exercise such as walking.

The following comprises the ideal exercise regimen for Blood Type A:

EXERCISE	DURATION	FREQUENCY
Hatha yoga	40–50 minutes	3–4 x week
T'ai Chi	40–50 minutes	3–4 x week
Aerobics (low impact)	40–50 minutes	2–3 x week
Treadmill	30 minutes	2–3 x week
Pilates	40–50 minutes	3–4 x week
Weight training (5–10 lb free weights)	15 minutes	2–3 x week

EXERCISE	DURATION	FREQUENCY
Cycling (recumbent bike)	30 minutes	2–3 x week
Swimming	30 minutes	2–3 x week
Brisk walking	45 minutes	2–3 x week

3 Steps to Effective Exercise

1. Warm up with stretching and flexibility moves before you start your aerobic exercise.
2. To achieve maximum cardiovascular benefits, work toward an elevated heart rate that is about 70 percent of your capacity. Once you reach the elevated rate, continue exercising to maintain that rate for twenty to thirty minutes. To calculate your maximum heart rate and performance level:
   - Subtract your age from 220.
   - Multiply the difference by .70 (or .60 if you are over age sixty). This is the high end of your performance.
   - Multiply the remainder by .50. This is the low end of your performance.
3. Finish each aerobic session with at least a five-minute cooldown of stretching and relaxation moves.

Getting Started: The First Month

IF YOU ARE NEW to the Blood Type Diet, the following guidelines will introduce you to the Blood Type O regimen over a period of one month. Follow these recommendations as closely as possible, using a notebook to record your personal experiences with the diet. In addition to factors that are measurable in laboratory tests, take the time to note changes in your energy levels, allergy symptoms, sleep patterns, digestion, and overall well-being.

Blood Type A Allergy Diet Checklist

Avoid or limit animal protein. Low levels of hydrochloric acid ☐
and intestinal alkaline phosphatase make it difficult for Blood
Type A to fully digest animal protein.

Derive your primary protein from soy foods and other plant ☐
proteins.

Include regular portions of richly oiled cold-water fish every ☐
week.

Include modest amounts of cultured dairy foods in your diet, ☐
but avoid fresh milk products, which cause excess mucus
production and can trigger inflammation.

Emphasize beans and legumes; beans provide an essential ☐
high-protein vegetable source for Blood Type A.

Don't overdo the grains, especially wheat-derived foods. ☐

Eat lots of BENEFICIAL fruits and vegetables, especially those ☐
high in antioxidants and fiber.

Drink green tea every day for extra immune system benefits ☐
and allergy-blocking compounds.

Week 1

Blood Type Diet and Supplements

- Eliminate your most harmful AVOID foods—red meat, most dairy, and negative lectin-containing nuts, beans, and seeds.

- Include your most important BENEFICIAL foods frequently throughout the
week. For example, have soy-based foods 5 times, and omega-3-rich fish 3
to 4 times, with lots of BENEFICIAL vegetables and fruit.

- Incorporate at least 1 SUPER BENEFICIAL into your daily diet. For example,
have a bowl of cherries as a snack, or a spinach salad with walnuts.

- If you have allergies, avoid whole-wheat products.

- Drink 2 to 3 cups of green tea every day.

Exercise Regimen

- Plan to exercise at least 4 days this week, for 45 minutes each day.

  2 days: walking or light aerobic activity

  2 days: Hatha yoga or T'ai Chi

- If you are ill or have low energy, start slowly, and gradually increase your duration and intensity of activity. The important factor is consistency. Just do it—as much as you're able.

- Use your journal to detail the time, activity, distance, and amount of weight lifted. Note the number of repetitions for each exercise.

▪ WEEK 1 SUCCESS STRATEGY ▪
Reduce Mucus

If you're overproducing mucus, the following tips can help you stay clear:

- Avoid dairy products. These can be mucus-producing for Type A.
- Begin your day by squeezing the juice of half a fresh lemon into a glass of water.
- Inhale steam from a bowl of hot water to clear your sinuses.
- Drink echinacea or lemon tea.

Week 2

Blood Type Diet and Supplements

- Begin to eliminate the next level of AVOID foods—grains, vegetables, and fruits that react poorly with Type A blood.

- Eat 2 to 3 BENEFICIAL proteins every day, with special emphasis on soy. Eat omega-3-rich fish at least 3 times a week.

- Continue to incorporate SUPER BENEFICIAL foods into your daily diet.

- Choose the NEUTRAL foods listed as "allowed frequently" over those listed "allowed infrequently."

- Manage your mealtimes to aid proper digestion. Avoid eating on the run. Make your meals relaxing, sit-down affairs. Eat slowly and chew thoroughly to encourage digestive secretions.

Exercise Regimen

- Continue to exercise at least 4 days this week, for 45 minutes each day.

  2 days: walking or light aerobic activity

  2 days: Hatha yoga or T'ai Chi

- If your work is sedentary, get in the habit of taking a couple of "movement" breaks during the day. Walk around the block or up and down stairs.

▪ WEEK 2 SUCCESS STRATEGY ▪
Help for the Sulfite-Sensitive

Sulfites are a commonly used preservative found in foods, alcoholic drinks (especially wines), and even in medications. Many consumers of the standard American diet experience severe allergy symptoms, including headaches, asthma, and even seizures from sulfites. The following foods and drugs may contain sulfites, according to the Food and Drug Administration. Not all manufacturers use sulfites in these products, and the amounts may vary. Remember to check the product label.

Alcoholic beverages	beer, cocktail mixes, wine, wine coolers
Baked goods	cookies, crackers, mixes with dried fruits or vegetables, pie crust, pizza crust, quiche crust, flour tortillas
Beverage bases	dried citrus fruit beverage mixes
Condiments and relishes	horseradish, onion and pickle relishes, pickles, olives, salad dressing mixes, wine vinegar
Confections, sweet sauces, and frostings	brown, raw, powdered, or white sugar derived from sugar beets; shredded coconut; corn syrup; maple syrup; fruit toppings; pancake syrup
Modified dairy products	filled milk (a specially prepared skim milk in which vegetable oils, rather than animal fats, are added to increase its fat content)

Drugs	anti-nausea drugs, cardiovascular drugs, antibiotics, tranquilizers, intravenous muscle relaxants, analgesics, seroids, asthma medications
Fish and shellfish	canned clams; fresh, frozen, canned, or dried shrimp; frozen lobster; scallops; dried cod
Fresh fruit and vegetables	sulfite use banned, except for fresh potatoes
Gelatins, puddings, and fillings	fruit fillings, flavored and unflavored gelatin, pectin, jelling agents, jams and jellies
Grain products and pastas	cornstarch, modified food starch, spinach pasta, gravies, hominy, breadings, batters, noodle/rice mixes
Plant protein products	soy protein
Processed foods	canned, bottled, or frozen fruit and fruit juices; dried fruit; vegetable juice; canned vegetables; pickled vegetables; dried vegetables; instant mashed potatoes; canned and dried soups

Week 3

Blood Type Diet and Supplements

- When you plan your meals for week 3, choose BENEFICIAL foods to replace NEUTRAL foods whenever possible. For example, choose tofu over chicken, or blueberries over an apple.
- Eliminate all remaining AVOID foods.
- Liberally incorporate SUPER BENEFICIAL foods into your daily diet.
- Drink 2 to 3 cups of green tea every day.

Exercise Regimen

- Continue to exercise at least 4 days this week, for 45 minutes each day.

  2 days: walking or light aerobic activity

  2 days: Hatha yoga or T'ai Chi

■ **WEEK 3 SUCCESS STRATEGY** ■
Conquering Chronic Ear Infections

Focus on preventive measures to avoid future ear infections. Blood Type A mothers, or mothers of Blood Type A infants, can start early by breast-feeding for a minimum of four months. Breast-feeding has shown a demonstrable effect in ear infection prevention. Conversely, formula feeding is associated with a greater risk for ear infections. If you use a bottle, avoid feeding while your child is lying on his or her back; this position greatly increases the likelihood of regurgitation of the bottle's contents into the middle ear.

Follow the recommended diet for your blood type while you are breast-feeding, even if your infant is a different blood type. When you begin the introduction of solid foods, start with easily digestible fruits and vegetables from your child's BENEFICIAL list. Delay the introduction of grains and legumes until the infant's digestive tract has developed stronger barrier mechanisms— preferably six to nine months.

Limit alcohol intake while breast-feeding, and maintain a no-smoking policy in your home.

Week 4

Blood Type Diet and Supplements

- Continue at the week 3 level, focusing on BENEFICIAL and SUPER BENEFICIAL foods.

Exercise Regimen

- Continue at the week 3 level.

- Review your progress, noting in your journal improvements in strength and flexibility. Determine which exercise regimen has worked for you, including time of day, setting, and activity level.

▪ **WEEK 4 SUCCESS STRATEGY** ▪
Detoxify

Toxins are the by-products of bacterial activity on unabsorbed foods that grow in your intestinal tract. Try this effective Blood Type A detoxification strategy for a week:

- One 250-mg capsule of dandelion (*Taraxacum officinale*) twice daily, or 2 to 3 cups of dandelion tea.
- 250 mg of milk thistle (*Silymarin*) daily.
- 1 tablespoon of fig powder in an 8-ounce glass of water daily.

A Final Word

IN SUMMARY, the secret to fighting allergies with the Blood Type A Diet involves:

1. Maximizing overall health by eating a diet rich in soy protein, BENEFICIAL seafood, and green vegetables.
2. Minimizing the consumption of pro-inflammatory lectins abundant in certain grains, beans, and vegetables that are not right for your blood type.
3. Regulating the effects of inflammatory molecules by avoiding red meat and high-fat foods.
4. Reducing stress and improving fitness by engaging in regular exercise appropriate for your blood type.
5. Using supplements to block the effects of pro-inflammatory lectins, provide antioxidant support, and balance immune function.

SIX

Blood Type

BLOOD TYPE B DIET OUTCOME: BREATHING FRESH AIR AGAIN
"I was at a point where I could not leave my apartment during cold weather, as I couldn't breathe cold air. Not great, since I live in Montreal. To date, my biggest advances are the following: one, no corn of any kind—improvement immediately in allergies; two, no chicken—each week I find myself more alert into the evening; three, I can exercise much more; and four, since beginning the diet, I've barely touched my inhaler."

BLOOD TYPE B DIET OUTCOME: VANISHING ALLERGIES
"I believe that by eliminating wheat from my diet, my lifelong nasal allergies have all but vanished. This alone is worth the price of admission! The day after I've eaten pasta or nonsprouted bread, I experience slight nasal congestion and drainage, but it goes away within a day if I don't continue eating wheat. In the past few weeks, I have begun to feel better than I have in years."

Self-reported outcomes from the Blood Type Diet Web site (www.dadamo.com)

Blood Type B: The Foods

THE BLOOD TYPE B Allergy Diet is specifically adapted for the prevention and management of allergies. A new category, **Super Beneficial,** highlights powerful disease-fighting foods for Blood Type B. The **Neutral** category has also been adjusted to de-emphasize foods that are less advantageous for you. Foods designated **Neutral: Allowed Infrequently** should be minimized or avoided entirely.

Your secretor status can influence your ability to fully digest and metabolize certain foods, so various adjustments in the values are made for non-secretors. If you do not know your secretor type, the odds are that you can safely use the "secretor" values, since the majority of the population (approximately 80 percent) are secretors. However, I urge you to get tested, since the variations are important for non-secretors who want to maximize the effectiveness of the Blood Type Diet. To find out how to get tested, visit our Web site (www. dadamo.com).

Blood Type B

TOP 10 ALLERGY-FIGHTING SUPER FOODS

1. Lean, organic, grass-fed red meat (especially lamb or muttton)
2. Richly oiled cold-water fish (halibut, sardines)
3. Cultured dairy (kefir, yogurt)
4. Flax (linseed) oil
5. Olive oil
6. Broccoli
7. Onion
8. Berries (cranberry, elderberry)
9. Turmeric
10. Green tea

The food charts are divided into three sections. The top of the chart suggests the average portion size and quantity per week or day, according to secretor status. These recommendations do *not* apply to the category **Neutral: Allowed Infrequently;** those foods should be eaten rarely, if at all. The charts also indicate differences in frequency for some foods based on ethnic heritage. It has been my experience that this factor has an impact upon the individual's ability to fully digest certain foods. For the purposes of blood type food choices, persons of Hispanic heritage should follow the guidelines for Caucasians, and American Native peoples should follow the guidelines for Asians.

The middle section of the chart gives the food values. The bottom section lists variants based on secretor status.

For your convenience, we have included a number of product names (Ezekiel 4:9 bread, Worcestershire sauce, etc.). However, keep in mind that commercial formulations vary among brands and regions. Even though a product may be listed as acceptable for you, always check its ingredients. Some products contain **Avoid** ingredients for your blood type. Of course, you may choose to make your own version of commercial products, such as bread and mayonnaise, using ingredients that suit your blood type. There are hundreds of delicious recipes for every blood type available on our Web site (www.dadamo.com) and in the book *Cook Right 4 Your Type: The Practical Kitchen Companion to Eat Right 4 Your Type.*

Meat/Poultry

Blood Type B is able to efficiently metabolize animal protein, but there are limitations that require careful dietary navigation. Chicken, one of the most popular food choices, disagrees with Blood Type B, because of a B-specific agglutinin, called a galectin, contained in the organ and muscle meat. This galectin can trigger inflammatory and autoimmune conditions. Turkey does not contain this lectin and can be eaten as an excellent alternative to chicken. Choose only the best quality (preferably free-range) chemical-, antibiotic-, and pesticide-free low-fat meats and poultry. Grass-fed cattle are far superior to grain-fed.

BLOOD TYPE B: MEATS/POULTRY

Portion: 4–6 oz (men); 2–5 oz (women and children)

	African	Caucasian	Asian
Secretor	3–6	2–6	2–5
Non-Secretor	4–7	4–7	4–7
	Times per week		

SUPER BENEFICIAL	BENEFICIAL	NEUTRAL: Allowed Frequently	NEUTRAL: Allowed Infrequently	AVOID
Goat Lamb Mutton	Rabbit Venison	Beef Buffalo Liver (calf) Ostrich Pheasant Turkey Veal		All commercially processed meats Bacon/ham/pork Chicken Cornish hen Duck Goose Grouse Guinea hen Heart (beef) Horse Partridge Quail Squab Squirrel Sweetbreads Turtle

Special Variants: *Non-Secretor* BENEFICIAL: liver (calf); NEUTRAL (Allowed Frequently): heart (beef), horse, squab, sweetbreads.

Fish/Seafood

Fish and seafood are an excellent source of protein for Blood Type B. Fish is a treasure trove of dense nutrients and is particularly BENEFICIAL for non-secretors. Seafood can be an excellent source of docosahexaenoic acid (DHA), a nutrient needed for proper nerve, tissue, and growth function. Richly oiled cold-water fish, such as halibut, mackerel, cod, and sardines, are excellent sources of anti-inflammatory omega-3 fatty acids. Do not waste your money on "farm-raised" fish: they have almost none of these precious oils.

BLOOD TYPE B: FISH/SEAFOOD

Portion: 4–6 oz (men); 2–5 oz (women and children)

	African	Caucasian	Asian
Secretor	4–5	3–5	3–5
Non-Secretor	4–5	4–5	4–5
	Times per week		

SUPER BENEFICIAL	BENEFICIAL	NEUTRAL: Allowed Frequently	NEUTRAL: Allowed Infrequently	AVOID
Cod	Caviar (sturgeon)	Abalone	Herring (pickled/smoked)	Anchovy
Halibut	Croaker	Bluefish	Salmon (smoked)	Barracuda
Mackerel	Flounder	Bullhead	Scallop	Bass (all)
Sardine	Grouper	Carp		Beluga
	Haddock	Catfish		Butterfish
	Hake	Chub		Clam
	Harvest fish	Cusk		Conch
	Mahi-mahi	Drum		Crab
	Monkfish	Gray sole		Crayfish
	Perch (ocean)	Halfmoon fish		Eel
	Pickerel	Herring (fresh)		Frog
		Mullet		Lobster
				Mussel
				Octopus

SUPER BENEFICIAL	BENEFICIAL	NEUTRAL: Allowed Frequently	NEUTRAL: Allowed Infrequently	AVOID
	Pike	Muskel-		Oysters
	Porgy	lunge		Pollock
	Salmon	Opaleye		Shrimp
	Shad	Orange		Snail (*Helix*
	Sole	roughy		*pomatia/*
	Sturgeon	Parrot fish		escargot)
		Perch		Trout (all)
		(silver/		Yellowtail
		white/		
		yellow)		
		Pompano		
		Red		
		snapper		
		Rosefish		
		Sailfish		
		Scrod		
		Scup		
		Shark		
		Smelt		
		Sole (gray)		
		Squid		
		(calamari)		
		Sucker		
		Sunfish		
		Swordfish		
		Tilapia		
		Tilefish		
		Tuna		
		Weakfish		
		Whitefish		
		Whiting		

Special Variants: *Non-Secretor* BENEFICIAL: carp; NEUTRAL (Allowed Frequently): barracuda, butterfish, caviar (sturgeon), flounder, halibut, pike, salmon, sole, snail (*Helix pomatia/*escargot), yellowtail; AVOID: scallop.

Dairy/Eggs

Dairy products, especially cultured dairy products, can be eaten by almost all Blood Type B secretors and to a lesser degree by non-secretors. Cultured dairy, such as yogurt and kefir, is particularly good for Blood Type B; these foods help build a healthy intestinal environment. Ghee (clarified butter) contains beneficial fatty acids believed to promote intestinal balance. Non-secretors should be wary of eating too much cheese, as they are more sensitive to many of the microbial strains in aged cheeses. This sensitivity is greater for those of African ancestry, but the sensitivity can also be found in Caucasian and Asian populations. Cheese consumption should also be limited for those who suffer from recurrent infections or allergies, as cheese can trigger inflammation and produce excess mucus. Eggs are a good source of DHA for Blood Type B and can be an integral part of the protein requirement. Do your best to find dairy products that are both hormone-free and organic.

BLOOD TYPE B: EGGS			
Portion: 1 egg			
	African	**Caucasian**	**Asian**
Secretor	3–4	3–4	3–4
Non-Secretor	5–6	5–6	5–6
		Times per week	

BLOOD TYPE B: MILK AND YOGURT			
Portion: 4–6 oz (men); 2–5 oz (women and children)			
	African	**Caucasian**	**Asian**
Secretor	3–5	3–4	3–4
Non-Secretor	1–3	2–4	1–3
		Times per week	

BLOOD TYPE B: CHEESE

Portion: 3 oz (men); 2 oz (women and children)

	African	Caucasian	Asian
Secretor	3–4	3–5	3–4
Non-Secretor	1–4	1–4	1–4
		Times per week	

SUPER BENEFICIAL	BENEFICIAL	NEUTRAL: Allowed Frequently	NEUTRAL: Allowed Infrequently	AVOID
Ghee (clarified butter) Kefir Yogurt	Cottage cheese Farmer cheese Feta Goat cheese Milk (cow/ goat) Mozzarella Paneer Ricotta	Camem- bert Casein Cream cheese Edam Egg (chicken) Emmenthal Gouda Gruyère Neufchâtel Parmesan Provolone Quark Sour cream	Brie Butter Buttermilk Cheddar Colby Half-and- half Jarlsberg Monterey Jack Muenster Sherbert Swiss cheese Whey	American cheese Blue cheese Egg (duck/ goose/ quail) Ice cream

Special Variants: *Non-Secretor* BENEFICIAL: whey; NEUTRAL (Allowed Frequently): cottage cheese, milk (cow); AVOID: Camembert, cheddar, Emmenthal, Jarlsberg, Monterey Jack, Muenster, Parmesan, provolone, Swiss cheese.

Oils

Blood Type B does best on monounsaturated oils and oils rich in omega series fatty acids. Olive oil fits the bill in both regards. Constituents in olive oil, such as flavonoids, squalenes, and polyphenols, act as powerful antioxidants. It should be used as the primary cooking oil.

Sesame, sunflower, and corn oils should be avoided, as they contain immunoreactive proteins that impair Blood Type B digestion.

BLOOD TYPE B: OILS			
Portion: 1 tblsp			
	African	Caucasian	Asian
Secretor	5–8	5–8	5–8
Non-Secretor	3–5	3–7	3–6
		Times per week	

SUPER BENEFICIAL	BENEFICIAL	NEUTRAL: Allowed Frequently	NEUTRAL: Allowed Infrequently	AVOID
Olive		Almond	Wheat germ	Avocado
		Black currant seed		Canola
		Cod liver		Castor
		Evening primrose		Coconut
		Flax (linseed)		Corn
		Walnut		Cottonseed
				Peanut
				Safflower
				Sesame
				Soy
				Sunflower

Special Variants: *Non-Secretor* BENEFICIAL: black currant seed, walnut.

Nuts/Seeds

Nuts and seeds can be an important secondary source of protein for Blood Type B. Walnuts are highly effective in inhibiting gastrointestinal toxicity; flax seeds contain beneficial immunity-enhancing chemicals. As with other aspects of the Blood Type B Diet plan, there are some idiosyncratic elements to the choice of seeds and nuts: Several, such as sunflower and sesame, have B-agglutinating lectins and should be avoided.

BLOOD TYPE B: NUTS/SEEDS			
Portion: Whole (handful); Nut Butters (2 tblsp)			
	African	**Caucasian**	**Asian**
Secretor	4–7	4–7	4–7
Non-Secretor	5–7	5–7	5–7
		Times per week	

SUPER BENEFICIAL	BENEFICIAL	NEUTRAL: Allowed Frequently	NEUTRAL: Allowed Infrequently	AVOID
Flax		Almond	Litchi	Cashew
Walnut (black)		Almond butter	Macadamia	Filbert (hazelnut)
		Beechnut	Pecan	Peanut
		Brazil nut		Peanut butter
		Butternut		Pignolia (pine nut)
		Chestnut		Pistachio
		Hickory		Poppy seed
		Walnut (English)		Pumpkin seed
				Safflower seed

SUPER BENEFICIAL	BENEFICIAL	NEUTRAL: Allowed Frequently	NEUTRAL: Allowed Infrequently	AVOID
				Sesame butter (tahini)
				Sesame seed
				Sunflower seed

Special Variants: *Non-Secretor* BENEFICIAL: walnut (English); NEUTRAL (Allowed Frequently): pumpkin seed.

Beans/Legumes

Blood Type B can do well on the proteins found in many beans and legumes, although this food category does contain more than a few beans with problematic lectins. Soy products should be de-emphasized, as they are rich in a class of enzymes that can interact negatively with the B antigen. Several beans, such as mung beans, contain B-agglutinating lectins and should be avoided.

BLOOD TYPE B: BEANS/LEGUMES			
Portion: 1 cup (cooked)			
	African	Caucasian	Asian
Secretor	5–7	5–7	5–7
Non-Secretor	3–5	3–5	3–5
		Times per week	

SUPER BENEFICIAL	BENEFICIAL	NEUTRAL: Allowed Frequently	NEUTRAL: Allowed Infrequently	AVOID
	Bean (green/ snap/ string)	Cannellini bean	Soy bean	Adzuki bean
		Copper bean		Black bean
				Black-eyed pea

SUPER BENEFICIAL	BENEFICIAL	NEUTRAL: Allowed Frequently	NEUTRAL: Allowed Infrequently	AVOID
	Fava (broad) bean Kidney bean Lima bean Navy bean Northern bean	Jicama bean Pea (green/ pod/ snow) Tamarind bean White bean		Garbanzo (chickpea) Lentil (all) Mung bean/ sprout Pinto bean Soy cheese Soy milk Soy, miso Soy, tempeh Soy, tofu

Special Variants: *Non-Secretor* NEUTRAL (Allowed Frequently): bean (green/snap/ string), fava (broad) bean, kidney bean, lima bean, navy bean, northern bean, soy milk; AVOID: soy bean.

Grains/Starches

Grains are a leading factor in triggering inflammatory and autoimmune conditions in Blood Type B. The wheat agglutinin is particularly harmful, as is the lectin found in corn. Non-secretors have an even greater sensitivity. Sprouted grains, such as those found in Essene bread (manna), are the exception. Sprouting makes the grains less reactive to the Type B immune system.

BLOOD TYPE B: GRAINS/STARCHES			
Portion: ½ cup dry (grains or pastas); 1 muffin; 2 slices of bread			
	African	Caucasian	Asian
Secretor	5–7	5–9	5–9
Non-Secretor	3–5	3–5	3–5
		Times per week	

SUPER BENEFICIAL	BENEFICIAL	NEUTRAL: Allowed Frequently	NEUTRAL: Allowed Infrequently	AVOID
	Essene bread (manna)	Barley	Rice flour/ products	Amaranth
	Ezekiel 4:9 bread	Quinoa	Soy flour/ products	Buckwheat
	Millet	Spelt flour/ products	Wheat (refined/ unbleached)	Cornmeal
	Oat bran		Wheat (semolina)	Couscous
	Oat flour		Wheat (white flour)	Grits
	Oatmeal			Kamut
	Rice (whole)			Popcorn
	Rice bran			Rice (wild)
	Rice cake			Rye
	Rice milk			Rye flour
	Spelt (whole)			Soba noodles (100% buck- wheat)
				Sorghum
				Tapioca
				Teff
				Wheat (whole)
				Wheat bran
				Wheat germ

Special Variants: *Non-Secretor* NEUTRAL (Allowed Frequently): amaranth, Ezekiel 4:9 bread, oat (all), rice (wild), sorghum, spelt (whole), tapioca; AVOID: soy flour/ products, wheat (all).

Vegetables

Vegetables can be your first line of defense against chronic disease. They provide a rich source of antioxidants and fiber and are essential to intestinal health. SUPER BENEFICIAL vegetables, such as maitake and shiitake mushrooms, are rich sources of antioxidants and immune modulators. Cabbage, cauliflower, and Brussels sprouts reduce the production of polyamines in the digestive tract. Onions and broccoli are potent detoxifiers. Broccoli contains allyl methyl trisulfide and dithiolthiones, which increase the activity of enzymes involved in detoxification, a function critical for Type Bs who want to control inflammation. Tomatoes contain a lectin that reacts with the saliva and digestive juices of Blood Type B secretors, although it does not appear to react with non-secretors. Corn has B-agglutinating activity and should be avoided.

An item's value also applies to its juice, unless otherwise noted.

BLOOD TYPE B: VEGETABLES			
Portion: 1 cup, prepared (cooked or raw)			
	African	Caucasian	Asian
Secretor Super/Beneficials	Unlimited	Unlimited	Unlimited
Secretor Neutrals	2–5	2–5	2–5
Non-Secretor Super/Beneficials	Unlimited	Unlimited	Unlimited
Non-Secretor Neutrals	2–3	2–3	2–3
			Times per day

SUPER BENEFICIAL	BENEFICIAL	NEUTRAL: Allowed Frequently	NEUTRAL: Allowed Infrequently	AVOID
Broccoli	Beet	Alfalfa sprouts	Potato	Aloe
Brussels sprouts	Beet greens	Arugula		Artichoke
Cabbage	Carrot	Asparagus		Corn
Cabbage (juice)*	Collards	Asparagus pea		Olive (all)
Cauliflower	Eggplant	Bamboo shoot		Pumpkin
Mushroom (maitake/ shiitake)	Kale	Bok choy		Radish/ sprouts
	Mustard greens	Carrot (juice)		Rhubarb
	Parsnip			Tomato

SUPER BENEFICIAL	BENEFICIAL	NEUTRAL: Allowed Frequently	NEUTRAL: Allowed Infrequently	AVOID
Onion (all)	Peppers (all) Potato (sweet) Yam	Celeriac Celery Chicory Cucumber Daikon radish Dandelion Endive Escarole Fennel Fiddlehead fern Horse-radish Kohlrabi Leek Lettuce (all) Mushroom (abalone/ enoki/ oyster/ porto-bello/ silver dollar/ straw/ tree ear) Okra Oyster plant Pickle (in brine or vinegar) Poi		

SUPER BENEFICIAL	BENEFICIAL	NEUTRAL: Allowed Frequently	NEUTRAL: Allowed Infrequently	AVOID
		Radicchio		
		Rappini (broccoli rabe)		
		Rutabaga		
		Scallion		
		Seaweeds		
		Shallot		
		Spinach		
		Squash (all)		
		Swiss chard		
		Taro		
		Turnip		
		Water chestnut		
		Watercress		
		Yucca		
		Zucchini		

Special Variants: *Non-Secretor* BENEFICIAL: okra; NEUTRAL (Allowed Frequently): artichoke, cabbage, eggplant, peppers (all), pumpkin, tomato; AVOID: potato.

*To obtain the benefits of cabbage juice, it must be consumed within one minute of juicing.

Fruits and Fruit Juices

Many SUPER BENEFICIAL fruits have powerful antioxidant effects, helping reduce infection that triggers inflammation. Watermelon supplies the antioxidant lycopene (which Blood Type B should eat in lieu of using tomatoes). Plums and prunes are high in the phytonutrients neochlorogenic and chlorogenic acids. These substances are classified as phenols, and their function as antioxidants has been well-documented. Cranberries are SUPER BENEFICIAL for Blood Type B individuals, especially non-secretors, who have a higher than average risk for urinary tract infections.

An item's value also applies to its juice, unless otherwise noted.

BLOOD TYPE B: FRUITS AND FRUIT JUICES

Portion: 1 cup

	African	Caucasian	Asian
Secretor	2–4	3–5	3–5
Non-Secretor	2–3	2–3	2–3
		Times per day	

SUPER BENEFICIAL	BENEFICIAL	NEUTRAL: Allowed Frequently	NEUTRAL: Allowed Infrequently	AVOID
Cranberry	Banana	Apple	Apricot	Avocado
Elderberry (dark blue/ purple	Grape	Blackberry	Asian pear	Bitter melon
	Papaya	Blueberry	Breadfruit	Coconut
		Boysen- berry	Cantaloupe	Persimmon
Pineapple		Canang melon	Currant	Pome- granate
Plum			Date	
Prune		Casaba melon	Fig (fresh/ dried)	Prickly pear
Water- melon		Cherry (all)	Honeydew	Star fruit (caram- bola)
		Christmas melon	Plantain	
		Crenshaw melon	Raisin	
		Dewberry		
		Goose- berry		
		Grapefruit		
		Guava		
		Kiwi		
		Kumquat		
		Lemon		

SUPER BENEFICIAL	BENEFICIAL	NEUTRAL: Allowed Frequently	NEUTRAL: Allowed Infrequently	AVOID
		Lime		
		Logan-berry		
		Mango		
		Mulberry		
		Muskmelon		
		Nectarine		
		Orange		
		Peach		
		Pear		
		Persian melon		
		Quince		
		Raspberry		
		Sago palm		
		Spanish melon		
		Strawberry		
		Tangerine		
		Young-berry		

Special Variants: *Non-Secretor* BENEFICIAL: blackberry, blueberry, boysenberry, cherry, currant, elderberry (dark blue/purple), fig (dried/fresh), guava, raspberry; NEUTRAL (Allowed Frequently): banana; AVOID: cantaloupe, honeydew.

Spices/Condiments/Sweeteners

Many spices are known to have medicinal properties. Turmeric improves liver function. Ginger is anti-inflammatory and aids digestive health, as does cayenne pepper. Licorice root provides antiviral support. Many common food additives, such as guar gum and carrageenan, enhance the effects of lectins found in other foods and should be avoided. Use caution when using prepared condiments. Often they contain wheat, which is a primary factor in the development of inflammatory conditions for Blood Type B.

SUPER BENEFICIAL	BENEFICIAL	NEUTRAL: Allowed Frequently	NEUTRAL: Allowed Infrequently	AVOID
Ginger	Horse-radish	Anise	Agar	Allspice
Licorice root*	Molasses (black-strap)	Apple pectin	Arrowroot	Almond extract
Pepper (cayenne)	Parsley	Basil	Chocolate	Aspartame
Turmeric		Bay leaf	Fructose	Barley malt
		Bergamot	Honey	Carra-geenan
		Caper	Maple syrup	Cinnamon
		Caraway	Mayon-naise	Cornstarch
		Cardamom	Molasses	Corn syrup
		Carob	Pickle (all)	Dextrose
		Chervil	Rice syrup	Gelatin (except veg-sourced)
		Chili powder	Sugar (brown/white)	
		Chive	Tamari (wheat-free)	Guarana
		Cilantro (corian-der leaf)	Vinegar (all)	Gums (acacia/Arabic/guar)
		Clove		Juniper
		Coriander		Ketchup
		Cream of tartar		Malto-dextrin
		Cumin		MSG
		Dill		Pepper (black/white
		Fenugreek		Soy sauce
		Garlic		
		Lecithin		
		Mace		
		Marjoram		

SUPER BENEFICIAL	BENEFICIAL	NEUTRAL: Allowed Frequently	NEUTRAL: Allowed Infrequently	AVOID
		Mint (all)		Stevia
		Mustard (dry)		Sucanat
		Nutmeg		Tapioca
		Oregano		
		Paprika		
		Pepper (pepper-corn/red flakes)		
		Rosemary		
		Saffron		
		Sage		
		Savory		
		Sea salt		
		Seaweeds		
		Senna		
		Tamarind		
		Tarragon		
		Thyme		
		Vanilla		
		Winter-green		
		Yeast (baker's/brewer's)		

Special Variants: *Non-Secretor* BENEFICIAL: oregano, yeast (brewer's); NEUTRAL (Allowed Frequently): stevia; AVOID: agar, fructose, pickle relish, sugar (brown/white).

*Not to be used if you have high blood pressure.

Herbal Teas

Several herbal teas can be SUPER BENEFICIAL allergy fighters for Blood Type B. Ginger contains pungent phenolic substances with pronounced antioxidative and anti-inflammatory activities. Sage is rich in rosmarinic acid, which acts to reduce inflammatory responses by altering the concentrations of inflammatory messaging molecules. The leaves and stems of the sage plant contain antioxidant enzymes, including superoxide dismutase (SOD) and peroxidase. When combined, these three components of sage—flavonoids, phenolic acids, and oxygen-handling enzymes—give it a unique capacity for stabilizing oxygen-related metabolism and preventing oxygen-based damage to the cells. Licorice root tea provides antiviral support for Blood Type B.

SUPER BENEFICIAL	BENEFICIAL	NEUTRAL: Allowed Frequently	NEUTRAL: Allowed Infrequently	AVOID
Ginger	Dandelion	Alfalfa	Dong quai	Aloe
Licorice root*	Ginseng	Burdock		Coltsfoot
Sage	Parsley	Catnip		Corn silk
	Peppermint	Chamomile		Fenugreek
	Raspberry leaf	Chickweed		Gentian
	Rosehip	Echinacea		Hops
		Elder		Linden
		Goldenseal		Mullein
		Hawthorn		Red clover
		Horehound		Rhubarb
		Mulberry		Shepherd's purse
		Rosemary		Skullcap
		Sarsaparilla		
		Senna		
		Slippery elm		

SUPER BENEFICIAL	BENEFICIAL	NEUTRAL: Allowed Frequently	NEUTRAL: Allowed Infrequently	AVOID
		Spearmint		
		St. John's wort		
		Strawberry leaf		
		Thyme		
		Valerian		
		Vervain		
		White birch		
		White oak bark		
		Yarrow		
		Yellow dock		
Special Variants: None.				

*Not to be used if you have high blood pressure.

Miscellaneous Beverages

Green tea should be part of every Blood Type B's health plan. It contains polyphenols, which enhance gastrointestinal health. Also, a compound in green tea, epigallocatechin gallate (EGCG), blocks receptors (IgE and histamine) involved in the allergic response. Avoid or limit alcohol to an occasional glass of wine. If you are a heavy coffee drinker, reduce your intake or eliminate it altogether.

SUPER BENEFICIAL	BENEFICIAL	NEUTRAL: Allowed Frequently	NEUTRAL: Allowed Infrequently	AVOID
Tea (green)			Beer	Liquor
				Seltzer

SUPER BENEFICIAL	BENEFICIAL	NEUTRAL: Allowed Frequently	NEUTRAL: Allowed Infrequently	AVOID
			Coffee (reg/decaf)	Soda (club)
			Tea, black (reg/decaf)	Soda (cola/diet/misc.)
			Wine (red/white)	

Special Variants: *Non-Secretor* BENEFICIAL: wine (red/white); NEUTRAL (Allowed Frequently): liquor, seltzer, soda (club); AVOID: coffee (reg/decaf), tea, black (reg/decaf).

Supplements

THE BLOOD TYPE B Diet offers abundant quantities of important nutrients, such as protein and iron. It is important to get as many nutrients as possible from fresh foods and use supplements only to fill in the minor deficiencies in your diet. The following supplement protocols are designed for Blood Type B individuals who are suffering from allergies or related conditions.

Note: If you are being treated for a medical condition, consult your doctor before taking any supplements.

Blood Type B
Immune System Health Maintenance

Use this protocol for 4–8 weeks, then discontinue for 2 weeks and restart.

SUPPLEMENT	ACTION	DOSAGE
Maitake extract (*Grifola frondosa*)	Modulates immune function	500 mg, 2–3 capsules, twice daily
L-arginine	Facilitates immune function and modulates nitric oxide synthesis	250 mg, 1–2 capsules, twice daily

SUPPLEMENT	ACTION	DOSAGE
Probiotic (preferably blood type–specific)	Promotes intestinal health	1–2 capsules, twice daily
High-potency vitamin-mineral complex (preferably blood type–specific)	Nutritional support	As directed
Sprouted food complex	Enhances detoxification	1–2 capsules, twice daily
Larch arabinogalactan	Promotes digestive and intestinal health	1 tblsp, twice daily, in juice or water

Blood Type B Specific Allergy Treatment Protocols

Use these protocols for 4–8 weeks, then discontinue for a week and restart. Protocols can be combined.

Anti-Inflammatory/Allergy Relief		
SUPPLEMENT	ACTION	DOSAGE
MSM (methylsulfo-nylmethane)	Has anti-inflammatory effects	500 mg, 1–2 capsules, twice daily
Quercetin	Has anti-inflammatory effects; liver protective	500 mg, twice daily, away from meals
Magnesium	Necessary for nerve and digestive health	650 mg, 1 capsule, twice daily
Green tea	Blocks pro-inflammatory receptors	1–3 cups daily

Sinus Relief		
SUPPLEMENT	ACTION	DOSAGE
Rosehips (*Rosa canina*)	Blocks histamine release	Solid extract: ¼ tsp, twice daily Tincture: 15 drops, twice daily
Magnolia flower (*Magnolia lilflora*)	Improves sinus and allergy symptoms	50 mg, 1–2 capsules, twice daily

SUPPLEMENT	ACTION	DOSAGE
Yerba santa (*Eriodictyon californicum*)	Helps eliminate congestion	Tincture: 10–15 drops, twice daily in warm water
Adrenal Support		
SUPPLEMENT	ACTION	DOSAGE
Schisandra/ Wu-Wei-Zi (*Schizandra chinensis*)	Supports nerve health; reduces stress	Tincture: 15–25 drops, twice daily
Spreading hogweed (*Boerhaavia diffusa*)	Acts as a stress modifier and liver protector; lowers cortisol	50–150 mg, twice daily
Licorice	Liver protective; enhances effects of naturally produced cortisone	Tea: 1–2 cups daily (remind of licorice potential for side effects)
Digestive System Repair		
SUPPLEMENT	ACTION	DOSAGE
L-glutathione	Acts as an anti-oxidant	100 mg, 1 capsule, twice daily
Thoroughwax/ Bei-Chai-Hu (*Bupleurum chinense*)	Improves intestinal health	500 mg, 1 capsule, twice daily
Quercetin	Has anti-inflammatory effects; liver protective	500 mg, twice daily, away from meals
Bromelain (pineapple enzyme)	Aids digestion	500 mg, 1–3 tablets, 4 times daily between meals, gradually decreasing
Larch arabinogalactan	Promotes digestive and intestinal health	1 tblsp, twice daily, in juice or water

The Exercise Component

FOR BLOOD TYPE B, stress regulation and overall fitness are achieved with a balance of moderate aerobic activity and mentally soothing, stress-reducing exercises. Below is a list of exercises that are recommended for Blood Type B.

EXERCISE	DURATION	FREQUENCY
Tennis	45–60 minutes	2–3 x week
Martial arts	30–60 minutes	2–3 x week
Cycling	45–60 minutes	2–3 x week
Hiking	30–60 minutes	2–3 x week
Golf (no cart!)	60–90 minutes	2–3 x week
Running or brisk walking	40–50 minutes	2–3 x week
Pilates	40–50 minutes	2–3 x week
Swimming	45 minutes	2–3 x week
Hatha yoga	40–50 minutes	1–2 x week
T'ai Chi	40–50 minutes	1–2 x week

3 Steps to Effective Exercise

1. Warm up with stretching and flexibility moves before you start your aerobic exercise.
2. To achieve maximum cardiovascular benefits, work toward an elevated heart rate that is about 70 percent of your capacity. Once you reach the elevated rate, continue exercising to maintain that rate for twenty to thirty minutes. To calculate your maximum heart rate and performance level:
   • Subtract your age from 220.
   • Multiply the difference by .70 (or .60 if you are over age sixty). This is the high end of your performance.
   • Multiply the remainder by .50. This is the low end of your performance.
3. Finish each aerobic session with at least a five-minute cool-down of stretching and relaxation moves.

Getting Started: The First Month

IF YOU ARE NEW to the Blood Type Diet, the following guidelines will introduce you to the Blood Type B regimen over a period of one month. Follow these recommendations as closely as possible, using a notebook to record your personal experiences with the diet. In addition to factors that are measurable in laboratory tests, take the time to note changes in your energy levels, allergy symptoms, sleep patterns, digestion, and overall well-being.

Blood Type B Allergy Diet Checklist

Eat small to moderate portions of high-quality, lean, organic meat (especially goat, lamb, and mutton) several times a week for strength, energy, and digestive health. ☐

Avoid chicken, which contains a highly allergenic lectin for Blood Type B. ☐

Include regular portions of richly oiled cold-water fish. Fish oils can help counter inflammatory conditions and balance immune activity. ☐

Regularly eat cultured dairy foods, such as yogurt and kefir, which are beneficial for digestive health. ☐

Eliminate wheat and corn from your diet—they produce allergic reactions for your blood type. ☐

Eat lots of BENEFICIAL fruits and vegetables. ☐

If you need a daily dose of caffeine, replace coffee with green tea. It isn't acidic and has substantially less caffeine than a cup of coffee. ☐

Avoid foods that are Type B red flags, especially chicken, corn, buckwheat, peanuts, soy beans, lentils, potatoes, and tomatoes. ☐

Week 1

Blood Type Diet and Supplements

- Eliminate your most harmful AVOID foods—chicken, corn, and wheat. The lectins in these foods can trigger inflammation.

- Include your most important BENEFICIAL foods on a regular schedule throughout the week. For example, have lean red meat 5 times, and omega-3-rich fish 3 to 5 times, with lots of BENEFICIAL vegetables and fruit.

- Incorporate at least 1 SUPER BENEFICIAL into your daily diet. For example, have a handful of walnuts as a snack, or eat yogurt mixed with berries for lunch.

- If you're a coffee drinker, begin to wean yourself by cutting your daily consumption in half, substituting green tea or a SUPER BENEFICIAL herbal tea.

Exercise Regimen

- Plan to exercise at least 4 days this week, for 45 minutes each day.

  2–3 days: aerobic activity

  1–2 days: Hatha yoga or T'ai Chi

- If you have severe allergy symptoms, start slowly and gradually increase your duration and intensity of activity. The important factor is consistency. Just do it—as much as you're able.

- Use your journal to detail the time, activity, distance, and amount of weight lifted. Note the number of repetitions for each exercise.

■ WEEK 1 SUCCESS STRATEGY ■
Neti Pots for Clear and Healthy Sinuses

Neti is the Ayurvedic and yoga practice of cleansing the nasal passages. Using a specially designed neti pot is a safe and effective way to perform this cleansing routine. A neti pot is a small pot with a spout that fits into the nostril and seals it.

- Fill the pot with lukewarm water and dissolve a teaspoon of ordinary salt (not sea salt) in the water.
- Stand over a sink, placing the spout against one nostril, so that it fits tightly. Lean forward, breathe relaxed through the mouth, and turn the head to one side. The water will flow by itself, in through one nostril and out of the other.

- When half of the water has run through one nostril, gently blow out any remaining water and mucus. Then repeat this process in the other nostril.
- After performing the process on both nostrils, bend forward and let your head hang loosely down, so that the remaining water can run out of the nose. Close one nostril with the index finger and turn the head alternating from side to side. Blow gently through one nostril at a time until the nose is dry.

There are a number of Internet sites that sell neti pots. You can also purchase them at yoga centers and at some health-food stores.

Week 2

Blood Type Diet and Supplements

- Begin to eliminate the next level of AVOID foods—seeds, beans, and legumes that have negative lectin activity.
- Eat at least 2 to 3 BENEFICIAL animal proteins every day—such as lamb, yogurt, or seafood.
- Initially, it is best to avoid foods on the list NEUTRAL: Allowed Infrequently.
- Continue to incorporate SUPER BENEFICIAL foods into your daily diet.
- If you're a coffee drinker, continue to cut your coffee intake, replacing it with green tea or SUPER BENEFICIAL herbal teas.

Exercise Regimen

- Continue to exercise at least 4 days this week, for 45 minutes each day.

  2–3 days: aerobic activity

  1–2 days: Hatha yoga or T'ai Chi

- If your work is sedentary, get in the habit of taking a couple of "movement" breaks during the day. Walk around the block or up and down stairs.

▪ WEEK 2 SUCCESS STRATEGY ▪
Search and Destroy Hidden Allergens

If you are sensitive to airborne allergens, here are some tips that go beyond the obvious:

- *Remove the carpet.* While the presence of a pet will bring that specific allergen into your home, carpeting has been found to significantly increase the concentration of the pet allergen.

- *Close the window.* If you're tempted to "air out" your house by flinging open the windows, think again. It's more likely that you'll invite the allergens inside.

- *Mop, don't vacuum.* Researchers have concluded that vacuuming in homes with cats substantially increases exposure to cat allergen—even when you use a HEPA filter.

- *Look under the hood.* Check under the hood of your car. If it is full of dirt and grime, clean it, because it is a harboring place for all sorts of allergens or irritants.

- *Watch out for flying food.* Particles of food can get into the air when you're cooking. Stay out of restaurants featuring foods that trigger allergies.

Week 3

Blood Type Diet and Supplements

- When you plan your meals for week 3, choose BENEFICIAL foods to replace NEUTRAL foods whenever possible. For example, choose lamb over beef, or blueberries over an apple.
- Eliminate all remaining AVOID foods.
- Liberally incorporate SUPER BENEFICIAL foods into your daily diet.

Exercise Regimen

- Continue to exercise at least 4 days this week, for 45 minutes each day.

  2–3 days: aerobic activity

  1–2 days: Hatha yoga or T'ai Chi

■ **WEEK 3 SUCCESS STRATEGY** ■
Visualize Your Way to a Better Immune System

Take advantage of Blood Type B's natural ability to relieve stress through meditation or guided imagery. I've never medicated Type B individuals who have high blood pressure without first teaching them some simple visualization techniques and sending them home to try them out for a few weeks. Those that did almost never required medication.

Here is a very simple visualization exercise to help control high blood pressure. Do this visualization two to four times daily for five to eight minutes.

Find a quiet place and make yourself comfortable and relaxed. Close your eyes and let your arms and hands lie limply at your sides or in your lap. Take a few deep breaths, inhaling through your nose and exhaling through your mouth, while imagining the red blood cells of your circulatory system coursing through your arteries and veins. See them slipping and sliding along the walls, which periodically open up like Venetian blinds to allow cells to move from the inside of the arteries out and from the outside in. Imagine the walls of your arteries relaxing and bending. Now expand the image and visualize your entire body. See the blood circulating from your heart to the arteries, to the capillaries, to the veins, then back to the lungs and heart.

Week 4

Blood Type Diet and Supplements

- Continue at the week 3 level, focusing on BENEFICIAL and SUPER BENEFICIAL foods.
- Evaluate the first 3 weeks, and make adjustments.

Exercise Regimen

- Continue at the week 3 level.
- Review your progress, noting in your journal improvements in strength and flexibility. Determine which exercise regimen has worked for you, including time of day, setting, and activity level.

▪ WEEK 4 SUCCESS STRATEGY ▪
Food Safety First

- Take this added measure before cooking meat or fish: Bring a pot of water to a boil. Turn off the water and let meat or fish soak for three to five minutes. This will help remove any chemicals and kill bacteria. Then, be sure to cook meat and fish thoroughly.

- Make sure hamburger is cooked thoroughly to an internal temperature of 160° F. The meat should be brown and the juice clear.

- If you have a cold or infection, avoid preparing or serving food to others.

- Use a vegetable/fruit wash to clean the skin and outer surface of fruits and vegetables before you slice into them.

- Wash your hands with warm soapy water between contact with raw meat and all other foods, including cooked meat.

A Final Word

IN SUMMARY, the secret to fighting allergies with the Blood Type B Diet involves:

1. Maximizing overall health by adhering to a high-protein diet that includes BENEFICIAL meat, seafood, and dairy.

2. Minimizing the consumption of pro-inflammatory lectins, most abundant in chicken and grains such as wheat, buckwheat, and corn.

3. Enhancing detoxification and elimination to increase liver efficiency and inhibit untoward provocation of the immune system by infectious agents.

4. Using supplements intelligently to block the effects of pro-inflammatory lectins, aid detoxification, provide antioxidant support, and balance immune function.

SEVEN

Blood Type

AB

BLOOD TYPE AB DIET OUTCOME: MULTIPLE BENEFITS

"The results are in. Weight Loss: fifteen pounds in the first month, after eliminating chicken and corn. Lifelong Acne: ended with elimination of chicken. Monthly Ear Infections: ended in first month. Hay Fever: eliminated after nine months on the diet. I now maintain my ideal weight (105 pounds) with no conscious effort on my part except to follow the diet, which is easy, because when I deviate my sinuses go crazy immediately."

BLOOD TYPE AB DIET OUTCOME: A BELIEVER

"I spent years with odd allergies of unknown origin. I tried endless changes in diet, cosmetics, and related personal products. Nothing seemed to work. I had rashes on my face and neck since the early 1970s, awful stomach upsets after meals, horrible gas, and various other body rashes and flare-ups. I made the following changes immediately after reading *Eat Right 4 Your Type*: gave up my heavy use of chicken and shrimp; began to eat only turkey and lamb; increased my use of soy, and got rid of all corn products. My rashes and stomach upsets have been gone from that point on! I didn't need much else to make me a believer."

Self-reported outcomes from the Blood Type Diet Web site (www.dadamo.com)

Blood Type AB: The Foods

THE BLOOD TYPE AB Allergy Diet is specifically adapted for the prevention and management of allergies. A new category, **Super Beneficial**, highlights powerful disease-fighting foods for Blood Type AB. The **Neutral** category has also been adjusted to de-emphasize foods that are less advantageous for you. Foods designated **Neutral: Allowed Infrequently** should be minimized or avoided entirely.

Your secretor status can influence your ability to fully digest and metabolize certain foods, so various adjustments in the values are made for non-secretors. If you do not know your secretor type, the odds are that you can safely use the "secretor" values, since the majority of the population (approximately 80 percent) are secretors. However, I urge you to get tested, since the variations are important for non-secretors who want to maximize the effectiveness of the Blood Type Diet. To find out how to get tested, visit our Web site (www.dadomo.com).

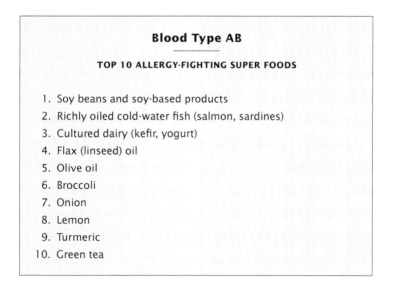

Blood Type AB

TOP 10 ALLERGY-FIGHTING SUPER FOODS

1. Soy beans and soy-based products
2. Richly oiled cold-water fish (salmon, sardines)
3. Cultured dairy (kefir, yogurt)
4. Flax (linseed) oil
5. Olive oil
6. Broccoli
7. Onion
8. Lemon
9. Turmeric
10. Green tea

The food charts are divided into three sections. The top of the chart suggests the average portion size and quantity per week or day, according to secretor status. These recommendations do *not* apply to the category **Neutral: Allowed Infrequently;** those foods should be eaten rarely, if at all. The charts also indicate differences in frequency for some foods based on ethnic heritage. It has been my experience that this factor has an impact upon the individual's ability to fully digest certain foods. For the purposes of blood type food choices, persons of Hispanic heritage should follow the guidelines for Caucasians, and American Native peoples should follow the guidelines for Asians.

The middle section of the chart gives the food values. The bottom section lists variants based on secretor status.

For your convenience, we have included a number of product names (Ezekiel 4:9 bread, Worcestershire sauce, etc.). However, keep in mind that commercial formulations vary among brands and regions. Even though a product may be listed as acceptable for you, always check its ingredients. Some products may contain **Avoid** ingredients for your blood type. Of course, you may choose to make your own version of commercial products, such as bread and mayonnaise, using ingredients that suit your blood type. There are hundreds of delicious recipes for every blood type available on our Web site (www.dadamo. com) and in the book *Cook Right 4 Your Type: The Practical Kitchen Companion to* Eat Right 4 Your Type.

Meat/Poultry

Blood Type AB is somewhat better adapted to animal-based proteins than Blood Type A, mainly because of the B gene's effects on the production of enzymes involved in fat transport and digestion. However, Type AB should limit meat and avoid chicken, which contains a B-immunoreactive lectin. Choose only the best quality (preferably free-range) chemical-, antibiotic-, and pesticide-free low-fat meats and poultry.

BLOOD TYPE AB: MEAT/POULTRY			
Portion: 4–6 oz (men); 2–5 oz (women and children)			
	African	Caucasian	Asian
Secretor	2–5	1–5	1–5
Non-Secretor	3–5	2–5	2–5
	Times per week		

SUPER BENEFICIAL	BENEFICIAL	NEUTRAL: Allowed Frequently	NEUTRAL: Allowed Infrequently	AVOID
	Lamb	Goat	Liver (calf)	All commercially processed meats
	Mutton	Ostrich		Bacon/ham/pork
	Rabbit	Pheasant		Beef
	Turkey			Buffalo
				Chicken
				Cornish hen
				Duck
				Goose
				Grouse
				Guinea hen
				Heart (beef)
				Partridge
				Quail
				Squab
				Squirrel
				Sweetbreads
				Turtle
				Veal
				Venison

Special Variants: *Non-Secretor* NEUTRAL (Allowed Frequently): quail, venison.

Fish/Seafood

Fish and seafood provide an excellent means of optimizing NK cell activity. Richly oiled cold-water fish, such as mackerel, salmon, and sardines, are good sources of omega-3 fatty acids. In general, many of the seafoods Blood Type AB must avoid have lectins with either A or B specificity or polyamines commonly found in the foods. Avoid consuming flash-frozen fish, which has high polyamine content.

BLOOD TYPE AB: FISH/SEAFOOD				
Portion: 4–6 oz (men); 2–5 oz (women and children)				
	African	Caucasian	Asian	
Secretor	4–6	3–5	3–5	
Non-Secretor	4–7	4–6	4–6	
		Times per week		

SUPER BENEFICIAL	BENEFICIAL	NEUTRAL: Allowed Frequently	NEUTRAL: Allowed Infrequently	AVOID
Mackerel	Cod	Abalone	Caviar	Anchovy
Salmon	Grouper	Bluefish	(sturgeon)	Barracuda
Sardine	Mahi-mahi	Bullhead	Mussel	Bass (all)
	Monkfish	Butterfish	Scallop	Beluga
	Pickerel	Carp	Squid	Clam
	Pike	Catfish	(calamari)	Conch
	Porgy	Chub	Whitefish	Crab
	Red	Croaker		Eel
	snapper	Cusk		Flounder
	Sailfish	Drum		Frog
	Shad	Halfmoon		Gray sole
	Snail (*Helix*	fish		Haddock
	pomatia/	Harvest		Hake
	escargot)	fish		Halibut
	Sturgeon			

SUPER BENEFICIAL	BENEFICIAL	NEUTRAL: Allowed Frequently	NEUTRAL: Allowed Infrequently	AVOID
		Herring (fresh)		Herring (pickled/ smoked)
		Mullet		Lobster
		Muskel-lunge		Octopus
		Opaleye		Oyster
		Orange roughy		Salmon (smoked)
		Parrot fish		Salmon roe
		Perch (all)		Shrimp
		Pollock		Sole
		Pompano		Trout (all)
		Rosefish		Whiting
		Scrod		Yellowtail
		Scup		
		Shark		
		Smelt		
		Sucker		
		Sunfish		
		Swordfish		
		Tilapia		
		Tilefish		
		Tuna		
		Weakfish		

Special Variants: *Non-Secretor* BENEFICIAL: herring (fresh); NEUTRAL (Allowed Frequently): trout (all).

Dairy/Eggs

Dairy products can be used with discretion by many Blood Type AB individuals, especially secretors. Some cultured dairy foods are especially BENEFICIAL, such as kefir and yogurt. Ghee (clarified butter) is an antioxidant, rich in omega-3 oils and short-chain fatty acids. Eggs, which, like fish, are a good source of docosahexaenoic acid, can complement the protein profile for your blood type. Do your best to find eggs and dairy products that are both hormone-free and organic.

BLOOD TYPE AB: EGGS

Portion: 1 egg

	African	Caucasian	Asian
Secretor	2–5	3–4	3–4
Non-Secretor	3–6	3–6	3–6
		Times per week	

BLOOD TYPE AB: MILK AND YOGURT

Portion: 4–6 oz (men); 2–5 oz (women and children)

	African	Caucasian	Asian
Secretor	2–6	3–6	1–6
Non-Secretor	0–3	0–4	0–3
		Times per week	

BLOOD TYPE AB: CHEESE

Portion: 3 oz (men); 2 oz (women and children)

	African	Caucasian	Asian
Secretor	2–3	3–4	3–4
Non-Secretor	0	0–1	0
		Times per week	

SUPER BENEFICIAL	BENEFICIAL	NEUTRAL: Allowed Frequently	NEUTRAL: Allowed Infrequently	AVOID
Ghee (clarified butter)	Cottage cheese	Casein	Cheddar	American cheese
Kefir	Egg (chicken)	Cream cheese	Colby	Blue cheese
Yogurt	Farmer cheese	Edam	Emmenthal	Brie
			Milk (cow)	Butter
			Monterey Jack	Buttermilk

SUPER BENEFICIAL	BENEFICIAL	NEUTRAL: Allowed Frequently	NEUTRAL: Allowed Infrequently	AVOID
	Feta	Egg	Sherbert	Camembert
	Goat	(goose/	Swiss	Egg (duck)
	cheese	quail)	cheese	Half-and-
	Milk (goat)	Gouda		half
	Mozzarella	Gruyère		Ice cream
	Ricotta	Jarlsberg		Parmesan
	Sour	Muenster		Provolone
	cream	Neufchâtel		
		Paneer		
		Quark		
		String		
		cheese		
		Whey		

Special Variants: *Non-Secretor* BENEFICIAL: ghee (clarified butter); NEUTRAL (Allowed Frequently): goat cheese, yogurt; AVOID: Emmenthal, Swiss cheese.

Oils

Olive oil, a monounsaturated fat, is SUPER BENEFICIAL for Blood Type AB. Constituents in olive oil, such as flavonoids, squalenes, and polyphenols, act as powerful antioxidants. It should be used as a primary cooking oil. Also SUPER BENEFICIAL is flax (linseed) oil, which is high in alpha-linolenic acid (ALA) and has anti-inflammatory properties.

Corn, sesame, and safflower oils can contain immunoreactive proteins that impair Blood Type AB digestion. These oils can interfere with proper immune function and stimulate the inflammatory response.

BLOOD TYPE AB: OILS			
Portion: 1 tblsp			
	African	**Caucasian**	**Asian**
Secretor	4–7	5–8	5–7
Non-Secretor	3–6	3–6	3–4
		Times per week	

SUPER BENEFICIAL	BENEFICIAL	NEUTRAL: Allowed Frequently	NEUTRAL: Allowed Infrequently	AVOID
Flax (linseed) Olive	Walnut	Almond Black currant seed Borage seed Canola Castor Cod liver Evening primrose Peanut Soy	Wheat germ	Coconut Corn Cottonseed Safflower Sesame Sunflower
Special Variants: None.				

Nuts/Seeds

Nuts and seeds can be an important secondary source of protein for Blood Type AB. Laboratory research has identified at least five natural phytochemicals in nuts that regulate the immune system and act as antioxidants. SUPER BENEFICIAL for Blood Type AB are flax seeds and walnuts, which are high in omega-3 fatty acids.

BLOOD TYPE AB: NUTS/SEEDS

Portion: Whole (handful); Nut Butters (2 tblsp)

	African	Caucasian	Asian
Secretor	5–10	5–10	5–9
Non-Secretor	4–8	4–9	5–9
		Times per week	

SUPER BENEFICIAL	BENEFICIAL	NEUTRAL: Allowed Frequently	NEUTRAL: Allowed Infrequently	AVOID
Flax	Chestnut	Almond	Brazil nut	Filbert (hazelnut)
Walnut (black/ English)	Peanut	Almond butter	Cashew	Poppy seed
	Peanut butter	Almond cheese	Cashew butter	Pumpkin seed
		Almond milk	Macadamia	Sesame butter (tahini)
		Beechnut	Pecan	Sesame seed
		Butternut	Pecan butter	Sunflower butter
		Hickory	Pistachio	Sunflower seed
		Litchi	Safflower seed	
		Pignolia (pine nut)		

Special Variants: *Non-Secretor* NEUTRAL (Allowed Frequently): peanut, peanut butter; AVOID: Brazil nut, cashew, cashew butter, pistachio.

Beans/Legumes

Blood Type AB does well on proteins found in many beans and legumes, although this food category contains more than a few beans with problematic A- or B-specific lectins. In general, soy beans and their related products are SUPER BENEFICIAL for the Blood Type AB immune system.

BLOOD TYPE AB: BEANS/LEGUMES			
Portion: 1 cup (cooked)			
	African	**Caucasian**	**Asian**
Secretor	3–6	3–6	4–6
Non-Secretor	2–5	2–5	3–6
		Times per week	

SUPER BENEFICIAL	BENEFICIAL	NEUTRAL: Allowed Frequently	NEUTRAL: Allowed Infrequently	AVOID
Soy bean	Lentil	Bean	Jicama	Adzuki bean
Soy cheese	(green)	(green/	bean	Black bean
Soy milk	Navy bean	snap/		Black-eyed
Soy, miso	Pinto bean	string)		pea
Soy,		Cannellini		Fava (broad)
tempeh		bean		bean
Soy, tofu		Copper		Garbanzo
		bean		(chickpea)
		Lentil		Kidney bean
		(domes-		Lima bean
		tic/red)		Mung bean/
		Northern		sprout
		bean		
		Pea		
		(green/		
		pod/		
		snow)		
		Tamarind		
		bean		
		White bean		

Special Variants: *Non-Secretor* NEUTRAL (Allowed Frequently): fava (broad) bean, navy bean, soy bean, soy (miso), soy (tempeh), soy (tofu); AVOID; jicama bean, soy cheese, soy milk.

Grains/Starches

Blood Type AB benefits from a moderate consumption of the proper grains for its blood type. Non-secretors should limit wheat. Blood Type AB is also sensitive to the lectin in corn and should avoid all corn flour products.

BLOOD TYPE AB: GRAINS/STARCHES			
Portion: ½ cup dry (grains or pastas); 1 muffin; 2 slices of bread			
	African	**Caucasian**	**Asian**
Secretor	6–8	6–9	6–10
Non-Secretor	4–6	5–7	6–8
		Times per week	

SUPER BENEFICIAL	BENEFICIAL	NEUTRAL: Allowed Frequently	NEUTRAL: Allowed Infrequently	AVOID
Essene bread (manna)	Amaranth Ezekiel 4:9 bread Millet Oat bran Oat flour Oatmeal Rice (whole) Rice (wild) Rice bran Rice cake Rye (whole) Rye flour/ products Soy flour/ products Spelt (whole)	Barley Couscous Quinoa Spelt flour/ products	Wheat (semo-lina) Wheat (whole) Wheat bran Wheat germ	Buckwheat Cornmeal Grits Kamut Popcorn Soba noodles (100% buckwheat) Sorghum Tapioca Teff Wheat (refined/ unbleached) Wheat (white flour)

Special Variants: *Non-Secretor* NEUTRAL (Allowed Frequently): Ezekiel 4:9 bread, spelt (whole); AVOID: soy flour/products, wheat (semolina), wheat (whole), wheat germ.

Vegetables

Vegetables can be your first line of defense against chronic disease. They provide a rich source of antioxidants and fiber and are essential to intestinal health. Blood Type AB SUPER BENEFICIALS include onions, which are high in quercetin, a flavonoid with potent anti-inflammatory properties, and other antioxidants that decrease oxidative stress and increase glutathione, which protects cells. Broccoli is a potent antioxidant. Mushrooms (maitake and the common domestic variety called silver dollar) are powerful infection fighters.

An item's value also applies to its juice, unless otherwise noted.

BLOOD TYPE AB: VEGETABLES			
Portion: 1 cup, prepared (cooked or raw)			
	African	**Caucasian**	**Asian**
Secretor Super/Beneficials	Unlimited	Unlimited	Unlimited
Secretor Neutrals	2–5	2–5	2–5
Non-Secretor Super/Beneficials	Unlimited	Unlimited	Unlimited
Non-Secretor Neutrals	2–3	2–3	2–3
	Times per day		

SUPER BENEFICIAL	**BENEFICIAL**	**NEUTRAL: Allowed Frequently**	**NEUTRAL: Allowed Infrequently**	**AVOID**
Broccoli	Alfalfa	Arugula	Daikon	Aloe
Cabbage	sprouts	Asparagus	radish	Artichoke
(juice)*	Beet	Asparagus	Olive	Corn
Cauli-	Beet	pea	(Greek/	Mushroom
flower	greens	Bamboo	green/	(abalone/
Mushroom	Carrot	shoot	Spanish)	shiitake)
(maitake/	(juice)	Bok choy	Poi	Olive (black)
silver	Celery	Brussels	Potato	Peppers (all)
dollar)	Collards	sprouts		
Onion (all)	Cucumber			

SUPER BENEFICIAL	BENEFICIAL	NEUTRAL: Allowed Frequently	NEUTRAL: Allowed Infrequently	AVOID
	Dandelion	Cabbage	Pumpkin	Pickles (all)
	Eggplant	Carrot	Taro	Radish/
	Kale	Celeriac		sprouts
	Mustard	Chicory		Rhubarb
	greens	Cucumber		
	Parsnip	(juice)		
	Potato	Endive		
	(sweet)	Escarole		
	Yam	Fennel		
		Fiddlehead		
		fern		
		Horse-		
		radish		
		Kohlrabi		
		Leek		
		Lettuce		
		(all)		
		Mushroom		
		(enoki/		
		oyster/		
		porto-		
		bello/		
		straw/		
		tree ear)		
		Okra		
		Oyster		
		plant		
		Radicchio		
		Rappini		
		(broccoli		
		rabe)		
		Rutabaga		
		Scallion		
		Seaweeds		

SUPER BENEFICIAL	BENEFICIAL	NEUTRAL: Allowed Frequently	NEUTRAL: Allowed Infrequently	AVOID
		Shallot		
		Spinach		
		Squash (all)		
		Swiss chard		
		Tomato		
		Turnip		
		Water chestnut		
		Watercress		
		Yucca		
		Zucchini		

Special Variants: *Non-Secretor* BENEFICIAL: tomato; NEUTRAL (Allowed Frequently): beet; AVOID: poi, taro.

*To obtain the benefits of cabbage juice, it must be consumed within one minute of juicing.

Fruits and Fruit Juices

Fruits are rich in antioxidants, and many, such as blueberries, elderberries, and cherries, contain pigments that inhibit intestinal toxins. Many fruits, such as pineapple, are rich in enzymes that can help reduce inflammation and encourage proper water balance. Grapes and grape juice are powerful antioxidants.

An item's value also applies to its juice, unless otherwise noted.

BLOOD TYPE AB: FRUITS AND FRUIT JUICES			
Portion: 1 cup			
	African	Caucasian	Asian
Secretor	3–4	3–6	3–5
Non-Secretor	1–3	2–3	3–4
		Times per day	

SUPER BENEFICIAL	BENEFICIAL	NEUTRAL: Allowed Frequently	NEUTRAL: Allowed Infrequently	AVOID
Cherry	Fig (fresh/	Apple	Apricot	Avocado
Cranberry	dried)	Blackberry	Asian pear	Banana
Grape (all)	Goose-	Blueberry	Breadfruit	Bitter melon
Lemon	berry	Boysen-	Canang	Coconut
Pineapple	Grapefruit	berry	melon	Dewberry
	Kiwi	Elderberry	Canta-	Guava
	Logan-	(dark	loupe	Mango
	berry	blue/	Casaba	Orange
	Plum	purple)	melon	Persimmon
	Water-	Grapefruit	Christmas	Pome-
	melon	(juice)	melon	granate
		Kumquat	Crenshaw	Prickly pear
		Lime	melon	Quince
		Mulberry	Currant	Sago palm
		Musk-	Date	Star fruit
		melon	Honeydew	(caram-
		Nectarine	Prune	bola)
		Papaya	Raisin	
		Peach	Tangerine	
		Pear		
		Persian		
		melon		
		Pineapple		
		(juice)		
		Plantain		
		Raspberry		
		Spanish		
		melon		
		Strawberry		
		Young-		
		berry		

Special Variants: *Non-Secretor* BENEFICIAL: blackberry, blueberry, elderberry, lime; NEUTRAL (Allowed Frequently): banana; AVOID: cantaloupe, honeydew, prune, tangerine.

Spices/Condiments/Sweeteners

Many spices have medicinal properties. Turmeric improves liver function. Ginger is anti-inflammatory and aids digestive health. Garlic improves immune health and is anti-inflammatory. Parsley contains quercetin, which is anti-inflammatory.

Many common food additives, such as guar gum and carrageenan, enhance the effects of lectins found in other foods and should be avoided.

SUPER BENEFICIAL	BENEFICIAL	NEUTRAL: Allowed Frequently	NEUTRAL: Allowed Infrequently	AVOID
Garlic	Horse-radish	Basil	Agar	Allspice
Ginger	Molasses (black-strap)	Bay leaf	Apple pectin	Amond extract
Parsley	Oregano	Bergamot	Arrowroot	Anise
Turmeric		Caraway	Chocolate	Aspartame
		Cardamom	Honey	Barley malt
		Carob	Maple syrup	Carra-geenan
		Chervil	Mayon-naise	Cornstarch
		Chili powder	Molasses	Corn syrup
		Chive	Rice syrup	Dextrose
		Cilantro (corian-der leaf)	Senna	Fructose
		Cinnamon	Soy sauce	Gelatin (except veg-sourced)
		Clove	Sugar (brown/white)	Guarana
		Coriander		Gums (acacia/Arabic/guar)
		Cream of tartar		Ketchup
		Cumin		Malto-dextrin
		Dill		
		Juniper		
		Licorice root*		

SUPER BENEFICIAL	BENEFICIAL	NEUTRAL: Allowed Frequently	NEUTRAL: Allowed Infrequently	AVOID
		Mace		MSG
		Marjoram		Pepper (black/ white)
		Mint (all)		
		Mustard (dry)		Pepper (cayenne)
		Nutmeg		
		Paprika		Pepper (pepper- corn/red flakes)
		Rosemary		
		Saffron		
		Sage		Pickles (all)
		Savory		Sucanat
		Sea salt		Tapioca
		Seaweeds		Vinegar (all)
		Stevia		Worcester- shire sauce
		Tamari (wheat- free)		
		Tamarind		
		Tarragon		
		Thyme		
		Vanilla		
		Winter- green		
		Yeast (baker's/ brewer's)		

Special Variants: *Non-Secretor* BENEFICIAL: bay leaf, yeast (brewer's); AVOID: agar, honey, juniper, maple syrup, rice syrup, sugar (brown/white).

*Do not use if you have high blood pressure.

Herbal Teas

Several herbal teas can be SUPER BENEFICIAL for Blood Type AB. Ginger contains pungent phenolic substances with pronounced anti-oxidative and anti-inflammatory activities. Echinacea is also a powerful antioxidant. Licorice root provides antiviral support.

SUPER BENEFICIAL	BENEFICIAL	NEUTRAL: Allowed Frequently	NEUTRAL: Allowed Infrequently	AVOID
Echinacea	Alfalfa	Catnip	Senna	Aloe
Ginger	Burdock	Chickweed		Coltsfoot
Licorice root*	Chamomile	Dong quai		Corn silk
	Dandelion	Elder		Fenugreek
	Ginseng	Goldenseal		Gentian
	Hawthorn	Horehound		Hops
	Parsley	Mulberry		Linden
	Rosehip	Peppermint		Mullein
	Strawberry leaf	Raspberry leaf		Red clover
		Sage		Rhubarb
		Sarsaparilla		Shepherd's purse
		Slippery elm		Skullcap
		Spearmint		
		St. John's wort		
		Thyme		
		Vervain		
		White birch		
		White oak bark		

SUPER BENEFICIAL	BENEFICIAL	NEUTRAL: Allowed Frequently	NEUTRAL: Allowed Infrequently	AVOID
		Yarrow Yellow dock		
Special Variants: None.				

*Do not use if you have high blood pressure.

Miscellaneous Beverages

A compound in green tea, epigallocatechin gallate (EGCG), blocks receptors involved in the allergic response (IgE and histamine). Coffee should be avoided by Type AB as it exacerbates allergies.

SUPER BENEFICIAL	BENEFICIAL	NEUTRAL: Allowed Frequently	NEUTRAL: Allowed Infrequently	AVOID
Tea (green)	Wine (red)	Seltzer Soda (club) Wine (white)	Beer	Coffee (reg/ decaf) Liquor Soda (cola/diet/ misc.) Tea, black (reg/ decaf)
Special Variants: *Non-Secretor* AVOID: beer.				

Supplements

THE BLOOD TYPE AB DIET offers abundant quantities of important nutrients, such as protein and iron. It is important to get as many nutrients as possible from fresh foods and use supplements only to fill in the minor deficiencies in your diet. The following supplement protocols are designed for Blood Type AB individuals who are suffering from allergies or related conditions.

Note: If you are being treated for a medical condition, consult your doctor before taking any supplements.

Blood Type AB
Immune System Health Maintenance

Use this protocol for 4–8 weeks, then discontinue for 2 weeks and restart.

SUPPLEMENT	ACTION	DOSAGE
Larch arabinogalactan	Promotes digestive and intestinal health	1 tblsp, twice daily, in juice or water
L-arginine	Facilitates immune function and increases nitric oxide synthesis	250 mg, 1–2 capsules, twice daily
Probiotic (preferably blood type–specific)	Promotes intestinal health	1–2 capsules, twice daily
High-potency vitamin-mineral complex (preferably blood type–specific)	Nutritional support	As directed
Sprouted food complex	Enhances detoxification	1–2 capsules, twice daily

Blood Type AB
Specific Allergy Treatment Protocols

Use these protocols for 4–8 weeks, then discontinue for a week and restart. Protocols can be combined.

Anti-Inflammatory/Allergy Relief		
SUPPLEMENT	ACTION	DOSAGE
Frankincense (*Boswellia serrata*)	Has anti-inflammatory effects	500 mg, 1–2 capsules, between meals

SUPPLEMENT	ACTION	DOSAGE
Magnolia flower (*Magnolia lilflora*)	Improves sinus and allergy symptoms	50 mg, 1–2 capsules, twice daily
Quercetin	Has anti-inflammatory effects; liver protective	500 mg, twice daily, away from meals
Green tea	Blocks pro-inflammatory receptors	1–3 cups daily

Sinus Relief		
SUPPLEMENT	ACTION	DOSAGE
Stone root (*Collinsonia canadensis*)	Supports sinus health	200 mg, 1–2 capsules, twice daily
Bromelain (pineapple enzyme)	Helps eliminate congestion; helps dissolve mucus	500 mg, 2–3 capsules daily
N-acetyl cysteine (NAC)	Helps eliminate congestion	200–500 mg, 1–2 capsules, twice daily

Digestive System Repair		
SUPPLEMENT	ACTION	DOSAGE
Bromelain (pineapple enzyme)	Aids digestion	500 mg, 1–3 tablets, 4 times daily between meals, gradually decreasing
Quercetin	Has anti-inflammatory effects; liver protective	500 mg, twice daily, away from meals
Chlorophyll	Detoxification agent	1–3 tsp daily
Larch arabinogalactan	Promotes digestive and intestinal health	1 tblsp, twice daily, in juice or water

Adrenal/Anti-Stress Support		
SUPPLEMENT	ACTION	DOSAGE
Tyrosine	Amino acid, helps balance dopamine/adrenaline axis	500 mg, twice daily

SUPPLEMENT	ACTION	DOSAGE
Ginseng, Siberian (*Eleuthero spp.*)	Great stress/ adrenal tonic	150–200 mg, once or twice daily

The Exercise Component

FOR BLOOD TYPE AB, overall fitness is achieved with a balance of moderate aerobic activity and mentally soothing, stress-reducing exercises. Below is a list of exercises that are recommended for Blood Type AB.

EXERCISE	DURATION	FREQUENCY
Martial arts	30–60 minutes	2–3 x week
Cycling	45–60 minutes	2–3 x week
Hiking	30–60 minutes	2–3 x week
Golf (no cart!)	60–90 minutes	2–3 x week
Walking	40–50 minutes	2–3 x week
Pilates	40–50 minutes	2–3 x week
Swimming	45 minutes	2–3 x week
Hatha yoga	40–50 minutes	1–2 x week
T'ai Chi	40–50 minutes	1–2 x week

3 Steps To Effective Exercise

1. Warm up with stretching and flexibility moves before you start your aerobic exercise.
2. To achieve maximum cardiovascular benefits, work toward an elevated heart rate that is about 70 percent of your capacity. Once you reach the elevated rate, continue exercising to maintain that rate for twenty to thirty minutes. To calculate your maximum heart rate and performance level:
   - Subtract your age from 220.

- Multiply the difference by .70 (or .60 if you are over age sixty). This is the high end of your performance.
- Multiply the remainder by .50. This is the low end of your performance.
3. Finish each aerobic session with at least a five-minute cooldown of stretching and relaxation moves.

Getting Started: The First Month

IF YOU ARE NEW to the Blood Type Diet, the following guidelines will introduce you to the Blood Type AB regimen over a period of one month. Follow these recommendations as closely as possible, using a notebook to record your personal experiences with the diet. In addition to factors that are measurable in laboratory tests, take the time to note changes in your energy levels, pain levels, sleep patterns, digestion, and overall well-being.

Blood Type AB Allergy Diet Checklist

Derive your protein primarily from sources other than red ☐ meat. Low levels of hydrochloric acid and intestinal alkaline phosphatase make it difficult for Blood Type AB to digest red meat.

Eliminate chicken and corn from your diet. They contain an ☐ immunoreactive lectin that is an allergen for Blood Type AB.

Eat soy foods and seafood as your primary protein. ☐

Include regular portions of richly oiled cold-water fish every ☐ week.

Include modest amounts of cultured dairy foods in your diet, ☐ but limit fresh milk products, which cause excess mucus production and can trigger inflammation.

Don't overdo the grains, especially wheat-derived foods. ☐
Avoid corn flour altogether.

Eat lots of BENEFICIAL fruits and vegetables, especially those ☐
high in antioxidants and fiber.

Avoid coffee. Substitute green tea every day for extra allergy- ☐
fighting benefits.

Week 1

Blood Type Diet and Supplements

- Eliminate your most harmful AVOID foods—chicken, corn, buckwheat, most shellfish, and lectin-activated beans.
- Avoid wheat if you have arthritis.
- Include your most important BENEFICIAL foods frequently throughout the week. For example, have soy-based foods 5 times, and omega-3-rich fish 3 to 4 times, with lots of BENEFICIAL vegetables and fruit.
- Incorporate at least 1 SUPER BENEFICIAL into your daily diet. For example, eat slices of fresh pineapple over yogurt, or sprinkle walnuts on a salad.
- If you're a coffee drinker, begin to wean yourself by cutting your daily consumption in half. Substitute green tea or 1 of the SUPER BENEFICIAL herbal teas.

Exercise Regimen

- Plan to exercise at least 4 days this week, for 45 minutes each day.

  2 days: walking or light aerobic activity

  2 days: Hatha yoga or T'ai Chi
- Use your journal to detail the time, activity, distance, and amount of weight lifted. Note the number of repetitions for each exercise.

▪ WEEK 1 SUCCESS STRATEGY ▪
Chi Breathing

Chi breathing is based upon the Taoist concept of Chi Gong, which represents energy as flowing according to certain routes in your body. Positive release is accessible through refining the breath. The calming, stress-relieving effects of this exercise are remarkable. It can be performed by anyone, regardless of age, fitness, or medical condition.

1. Stand comfortably, feet shoulder-width apart, knees slightly bent, arms at your side. Relax your neck and shoulder muscles and focus in on your solar plexus (center of the body). It is okay to sway a bit—that's normal.
2. Start to rock back and forth gently. Inhale deeply as you rock forward onto the balls of your feet; exhale as you rock backward onto your heels.
3. As you inhale, lift your relaxed arms up and forward, keeping them relaxed and slightly bent. As you exhale, let your arms float down. Imagine that your hands are pulsing around an imaginary ball of energy.
4. Repeat, gradually refining the rhythm and developing the ability to "drop" your breath from the lungs to the solar plexus.
5. Repeat four to five times, then relax, letting your hands drop to your sides and closing your eyes. Concentrate on feeling relaxed and centered.

Week 2

Blood Type Diet and Supplements

- Begin to eliminate the next level of AVOID foods—grains, vegetables, and fruits—that react poorly with Type AB blood.
- Eat 2 to 3 BENEFICIAL proteins every day.
- Continue to incorporate SUPER BENEFICIAL foods into your daily diet.
- Choose the NEUTRAL foods listed as "Allowed Frequently" over those listed "Allowed Infrequently."
- If you're a coffee drinker, continue to cut your coffee intake, replacing it with BENEFICIAL herbal teas. Drink a cup of green tea every morning.

- Manage your mealtimes to aid proper digestion. Avoid eating on the run. Make your meals relaxing, sit-down affairs. Eat slowly and chew thoroughly to encourage digestive secretions.

Exercise Regimen

- Continue to exercise at least 4 days this week, for 45 minutes each day.

  2 days: walking or light aerobic activity

  2 days: Hatha yoga or T'ai Chi

- If your work is sedentary, get in the habit of taking a couple of "movement" breaks during the day. Walk around the block or up and down stairs.

▪ WEEK 2 SUCCESS STRATEGY ▪
Wean Yourself from Coffee

If you're a regular coffee drinker, you're probably familiar with the symptoms that occur when you don't get your daily dose. Caffeine withdrawal can cause an excruciating headache, as well as drowsiness and irritability. In extreme cases, nausea and vomiting can occur. For this reason, cold turkey may not be the best way to break your coffee habit. Here's a gentler method.

1. Begin to slowly cut your intake, at the rate of half a cup every day or two.
2. Plan ahead to substitute a healthy hot drink for your usual cup of coffee. Green tea is an excellent replacement, and it has a small amount of caffeine. You can also substitute BENEFICIAL herbal teas.
3. If you're accustomed to taking an afternoon coffee break, go for a brisk walk instead.
4. As you reduce your coffee intake, also begin to drink less coffee per cup—by making a weaker blend or adding soy milk.
5. Get plenty of rest!

Week 3

Blood Type Diet and Supplements

- When you plan your meals for week 3, choose BENEFICIAL foods to replace NEUTRAL foods whenever possible.
- Eliminate all remaining AVOID foods.
- Liberally incorporate SUPER BENEFICIAL foods into your daily diet.
- Completely wean yourself from coffee, substituting green tea or herbal tea.

Exercise Regimen

- Continue to exercise at least 4 days this week, for 45 minutes each day.

  2 days: walking or light aerobic activity

  2 days: Hatha yoga or T'ai Chi

▪ WEEK 3 SUCCESS STRATEGY ▪
Reduce Mucus

If you're overproducing mucus, the following tips can help you stay clear:

- Avoid dairy products. These can be mucus-producing for Type AB.
- Begin your day by squeezing the juice of half a fresh lemon into a glass of water.
- Inhale steam from a bowl of hot water to clear your sinuses.
- Drink echinacea or lemon tea.

Week 4

Blood Type Diet

- Continue at the week 3 level, focusing on BENEFICIAL and SUPER BENEFICIAL foods.

Exercise Regimen

- Continue at the week 3 level.
- Review your progress, noting in your journal improvements in strength and flexibility. Determine which exercise regimen has worked for you, including time of day, setting, and activity level.

■ **WEEK 4 SUCCESS STRATEGY** ■
First, Cleanse the Bowels

Resolve to rid your body of any toxins that diminish your health. Toxins are the by-products of unabsorbed foods that grow in your intestinal tract. In my conservative estimation, at least 50 percent of all the illnesses I treat involve some sort of toxicity. Hippocrates, the father of modern medicine, knew the elemental importance of what he advised physicians in the treatment of their patients: "First, cleanse the bowels."

Follow these guidelines to detoxify:

- *Eat only those foods that are recommended for your blood type.* When you eat foods on the AVOID list, they are poorly digested and leave toxic by-products in your digestive tract.
- *Eat organic.* Chemicals, pollutants, and improper storage make foods harder to digest and leave toxins lingering in your digestive tract.
- *Eat natural.* Avoid artificial sweeteners, colors, and flavorings.
- *Eat fresh.* Limit your consumption of packaged, frozen, and canned foods.
- *Eat safe.* Avoid nitrates and nitrites—found in smoked, cured, and pickled foods.
- *Avoid fermented foods (cheese, beer, and yeast extracts), canned and frozen foods, and aged or sharp cheeses.* These foods are particularly high in proteins that are destructive to the intestinal tract.

A Final Word

IN SUMMARY, the secret to fighting allergies with the Blood Type AB Diet involves:

1. Maximizing overall health by eating a diet rich in soy protein, BENEFICIAL seafood, cultured dairy, and green vegetables.

2. Minimizing the consumption of pro-inflammatory lectins, most abundant in chicken and grains such as wheat, buckwheat, and corn.

3. Enhancing detoxification and elimination to increase liver efficiency and inhibit untoward provocation of the immune system by infectious agents.

4. Using supplements to block the effects of pro-inflammatory lectins, provide antioxidant support, and help balance immune function.

Appendices

A Simple Definition of Terms

agglutination: Clumping, or "gluing" together. One means by which the immune system defends against foreign matter and toxins, notably against lectins and opposing blood type material.

allergy: A sensitivity to a foreign substance introduced to the body, usually in the form of pollen or food, which triggers a defensive reaction of the body's immune system, producing large amounts of a special class of antibodies called immunoglobulin E (IgE).

antibody: The product of the immune system when it is stimulated by specific antigens. There are many classes of antibodies, among them "agglutinins," which isolate foreign substances by clumping them together so that they may be eliminated. Blood Types O, A, and B manufacture antibodies to other blood types. Blood Type AB, the universal recipient, manufactures no antibodies to other blood types.

antigen: A chemical that provokes an immune system antibody response. The blood type "ID" present on the blood cells, identified as Type A or B, is one example. A Type AB cell has both of these antigens. The blood type having no antigen is described as O, or "zero." As we age, it is to our advantage to shore up our store of circulating anti-blood–type antigens, as lower levels mean increased susceptibility to diseases arising from substances and organisms bearing opposing antigens.

antioxidant: A substance known to moderate the oxidation, or aging, process in human cells, by lowering free radical levels. Vitamins C and E and many plants and plant-derived substances such as green tea, quercetin, larch arabinogalactan, and milk thistle are potent antioxidants.

asthma: A reaction that constricts the airways and causes difficulty in breathing.

autoimmune disease: A disease generated when the cells that normally defend the body against infections mistakenly attack its own cells, tissues, and organs.

blood type: The term commonly used to refer to the ABO blood group system. Originally used primarily to determine suitable blood and organ donor–recipient matches, ABO type determines many of the digestive and immunological characteristics of the body, as well as susceptibility to the diseases arising from infection, immune suppression, and digestive impairment. It is also one of the tools of anthropology in establishing the origins, socioeconomic development, and movements of ancient peoples.

B-lymphocyte cells: White blood cells that create an immune response when activated by a foreign antigen. B-lymphocytes develop in the bone marrow and are responsible for the production of antibodies.

celiac disease: An intolerance to gluten that produces an inflammation of the intestinal lining. Inflammation and atrophy of the lining of the small intestine lead to impaired nutrient absorption.

complement: Proteins involved in the inflammatory response.

cytokines: Messenger proteins that induce the release of acute phase proteins, such as complement, and act as fever producers.

hay fever: An allergy syndrome, usually seasonally triggered by airborne pollens and mold spores. During the spring and fall, people with hay fever experience increased symptoms of sneezing, congestion, runny nose; and itchiness in the nose, roof of the mouth, throat, eyes, and ears.

histamine: A chemical released by immune cells during an allergic reaction and also during infection with viruses that cause the common cold. The interaction of histamine with the mucous membranes of the eyes and nose results in watery eyes and the runny nose often accompanying allergies and colds.

immune system: The physiological determination of and response to "self" and "non-self" accomplished through the action of many organs and cells throughout the body, essential to the preservation of its health and integrity.

immunoglobulin A (IgA): IgA is the antibody most involved in the health of the digestive system. It is the main antibody in a variety of secretions such as saliva, milk, and the mucus lining the airways and digestive tract.

immunoglobulin E (IgE): A special class of antibodies specific for allergens.

isohemagglutinins: Opposing ABO blood group antibodies.

lactose intolerance: An inherited inability to properly digest dairy foods, due to a deficiency in the amount of the enzyme lactase, which is normally produced by the cells that line the small intestine. Lactase breaks down milk sugar into simpler forms that can then be absorbed into the bloodstream. Symptoms of lactose intolerance include abdominal cramps, flatulence, and diarrhea.

leaky gut: A condition resulting when partially digested foods, toxins, and bad bacteria permeate the small intestine and enter the bloodstream.

lectins: Proteins that attach to preferred receptors in the human body. Food lectins are often blood type specific. A lectin's action may initiate agglutination, inflammation, the abnormal proliferation of cells of the immune and nervous systems, or insulin resistance, depending upon the type of cells targeted. Abundant in the vegetable kingdom, lectins are fewer in number and type among animal foods.

otitis media: An infection of the inner ear, most common in young children.

selectins: Proteins that mediate the binding of white blood cells to the walls of the blood vessels, signaling the initiation of the inflammatory response.

sinusitis: An acute or chronic inflammation of the nasal sinuses, which usually begins with a cold. People with allergies seem to be predisposed to developing sinusitis because the inflammation of the sinuses and nasal mucus lining prevents the sinus cavities from clearing the accumulated bacteria.

T-lymphocyte cells: White blood cells developed in the thymus that are responsible for cell-mediated immunity.

FAQs: Blood Type and Allergies

What is the difference between a food allergy and a food intolerance?

A true allergy is a response mounted by the immune system to a particular food, inhalant, or chemical. It involves an antibody reaction to a foreign antigen. An intolerance is a reaction that involves a different mechanism. For example, the problem some people have digesting the lactose in milk is not due to a lactose *allergy*. Rather, these individuals lack the specific enzyme needed to break it down. They are lactose *intolerant*.

I am quite allergic to the sulfites that are used as preservatives in many foods. Do you have any suggestions?

The obvious solution is to stay away from them! Then the trace mineral molybdenum might help. Molybdenum functions as a component in several enzymes, including those involved in alcohol detoxification, uric acid formation, and sulfur metabolism. In one study, molybdenum supplementation brought about complete resolution of symptoms of sulfite toxicity, such as increased heart rate, shortness of breath, headache, disorientation, nausea, and vomiting. There is no official recommended dietary allowance (RDA) for molybdenum, but the estimated range recommended by the Food and Nutrition Board as safe and adequate is 75 to 250 mcg per day for adults.

I appear to be allergic to a food that is BENEFICIAL for my blood type. What should I do?

Don't eat it. In the event that your body chemistry has been altered by drugs, surgery, or disease, you may have different tolerances for food. The best thing to do in this situation is avoid the allergic foods and the AVOIDS for your blood type. Choose as many BENEFICIAL and NEUTRAL foods as possible. This sensitivity may change over time.

I am Type AB, and peanuts are listed as BENEFICIAL for me. Is aflatoxin a problem?

Peanuts and peanut butter are required to be inspected specifically for aflatoxin. It is no longer believed to be a concern in commercial preparations. It may be a problem if small private growers sell moldy nuts directly to small buyers, like health-food stores, for sale as is or as peanut butter.

Should I avoid genetically engineered food?

Yes! Genetic engineering moves lectin molecules from one species to another. Since lectins are the molecules that interact with our blood types, a normally BENEFICIAL food can easily become an AVOID. Currently, the only way to safely avoid genetically engineered foods is to eat organic.

Are there foods that can help the growth of beneficial bacteria? I'm Blood Type O.

I recommend the daily consumption of probiotics (a term that means "in favor of life"). Probiotics, including lactic acid bacteria and their fermented (cultured) food products, are known to decrease IgE-mediated responses, inactivate and eliminate carcinogens, produce digestive enzymes that help digest proteins, carbohydrates, and fibers, decrease intestinal permeability, decrease food sensitivities, and enhance liver function.

You can improve the action of probiotics when they are blood type–specific. Blood type antigens are prominent in your digestive tract and, if you are a secretor, also in the mucus that lines your digestive tract. Many of the bacteria in your digestive tract use your blood type as a preferred food supply. In fact, blood type specificity is common among intestinal bacteria, with almost one-half of strains tested showing some Blood Type A, B, or O specificity. See appendix C for information about blood type–specific products, including probiotics.

What is your opinion of allergy "scratch" tests?

They are very unreliable as a diagnostic tool for detecting food allergies. Usually these tests will not help diagnose nonclassic reactions—such as lectin reactions—which are much more common than classic allergies.

How can it be that wheat isn't good for anyone? Hasn't it been a staple in our diet for thousands of years?

Wheat as we know it today is not the same as it was at the very beginning. The wheat that we eat now has a protein content as high as 13 percent, versus the more ancient wheat varieties, which had a protein content of about 2 percent. Increasing the protein content has had the effect of making wheat a viable source of protein for many people around the world but has also increased the allergenic (gliandin, gluten, and lectin containing), pro-inflammatory, and metabolic-blocking portions of the plant almost sevenfold.

Aside from the under-investigated metabolic effects of wheat lectin, classic hypersensitivity to wheat is found in many infants and adults. Reactions are often localized in the GI tract. In a study of asthmatic patients, 46 percent of children and 34 percent of adults were found to have IgE to wheat. In another study, specificity for wheat allergen using the same system was 98 percent. Wheat allergy was found to cause a persistent food hypersensitivity in atopic dermatitis patients (75 percent remained intolerant). In 102 grass-pollen allergic children, 12 percent were found to be allergic to wheat.

My Type A child has frequent ear infections. Besides diet, are there any suggestions for relieving her symptoms?

In a recently published study, mullein/garlic eardrops were shown to work as well as antibiotic therapy in relieving symptoms. However, if your child has chronic ear infections, there is probably a strong dietary correlation. Begin to eliminate the foods listed as AVOID for Blood Type A, and you should see a reduction in infections. Many of my patients have eliminated ear infections completely simply by following the diet.

I am Blood Type B. Are there specific correlations between migraine headaches and blood type?

Migraine headaches are often the result of food reactions. In particular, foods containing nitrites (smoked fish, frankfurters, bacon, bologna, etc.) as preservatives can trigger headaches. The flavor enhancer monosodium glutamate (MSG) can trigger headaches. Many food additives enhance the effects of lectins in your system. My best advice is to adhere to the right diet for your blood type.

Why does smoking or curing foods produce nitrates or nitrites?

Nitrate (NO_3) is a naturally occurring form of nitrogen found in soil. Nitrogen is essential to all life, and most crop plants require large quantities to sustain high yields. The formation of nitrates is an integral part of the nitrogen cycle in our environment. In moderate amounts, nitrate is a harmless constituent of food and water. Nitrites are thought to be problematic because they can be converted into nitrosamine compounds with known carcinogenicity. Nitrates and nitrites are compounds typically found in smoked or cured meats, though they can be present in many vegetables as well. The main significance of nitrites and nitrates is that they may be linked to cancer of the stomach.

APPENDIX C

Resources
and Products

General

Food Allergy and Anaphylaxis Network
10400 Eaton Place, Suite 107
Fairfax, VA 22030
1-800-929-4040
http://www.foodallergy.org

American College of Allergy, Asthma and Immunology
85 W. Algonquin Road, Suite 550
Arlington Heights, IL 60005
1-800-842-7777
http://allergy.mcg.edu

Asthma and Allergy Foundation of America
1125 15th Street, N.W., Suite 502
Washington, DC 20036
1-800-7-ASTHMA
http://www.aafa.org

American Academy of Allergy,
Asthma and Immunology (AAAAI)
611 East Wells Street
Milwaukee, WI 53202
1-800-822-ASMA (2762)
http://www.aaaai.org

Joint Council of Allergy, Asthma, and Immunology
50 N. Brockway, Suite 33
Palatine, IL 60067
847-934-1918
http://www.jcaai.org

National Allergy Bureau
AAAAI Executive Office
555 East Wells Street
Milwaukee, WI 53202-3823
414-272-6071 or 1-800-POLLEN
nab@aaaai.org

Nutrition Research
The Institute for Human Individuality
Southwest College of Naturopathic Medicine
2140 E. Broadway Road
Tempe, AZ 85282
480-858-9100
www.ifhi-online.org

The Institute for Human Individuality is under the 501c3 status of Southwest College of Naturopathic Medicine. Its prime goal is to foster research in the expanding area of human nutrigenomics. Nutrigenomics seeks to provide a molecular understanding for how common dietary chemicals affect health by altering the expression or structure of an individual's genetic makeup. (IFHI is currently conducting a twelve-week randomized, double-blind, controlled trial implementing the Blood Type Diet to determine its effects on the outcomes of patients with rheumatoid arthritis.)

Blood Type–Specific Resources

Dr. Peter D'Adamo

The D'Adamo Clinic in Wilton, Connecticut, blends time-honored natural healing techniques with state-of-the-art diagnostics. The clinic staff is comprised of naturopathic physicians (N.D.s) working with medical doctors (M.D.s), nurses (R.N.s), and other licensed health professionals, all under the precepts and guidance of Dr. Peter D'Adamo. To find out more or to schedule an appointment, please contact:

The D'Adamo Clinic, LLC
213 Danbury Road
Wilton, CT 06897
203-834-7500

www.dadamo.com

The World Wide Web has proven to be a valuable venue for exploring and applying the tenets of the Blood Type Diet and lifestyle. Since January 1997, hundreds of thousands have visited the site to participate in the ABO chat groups, to peruse the scientific archives, to share experiences and recipes, and to learn more about the science of blood type.

Blood Type Specialty Products and Supplements

North American Pharmacal, Inc., is the official distributor of Blood Type specialty products. The product line includes supplements, books, tapes, teas, meal replacement bars, cosmetics, and support material that make eating and living right for your type easier.

North American Pharmacal, Inc.
12 High Street
Norwalk, CT 06851
Tel: 203-866-7664
Fax: 203-838-4066
Toll free: 877-ABO TYPE (877-226-8973)
www.4yourtype.com

Home Blood-Typing Kits

North American Pharmacal, Inc., is the official distributor of Home Blood Type Testing Kits. Each kit costs $9.95 (plus shipping and handling) and is a single-use, disposable, educational device capable of determining one individual's ABO and Rhesus (Rh) blood type. Results are obtained within about four to five minutes. If you have several friends or family members who need to learn their blood type, you will need to order a separate home blood-typing kit for each individual.

The Blood Type Library

The following books are available in bookstores, health-food stores, selected grocery and specialty stores, on the Web, and through North American Pharmacal.

Eat Right 4 Your Type
The Individualized Diet Solution to Staying Healthy, Living Longer, and Achieving Your Ideal Weight
By Dr. Peter J. D'Adamo, with Catherine Whitney
G. P. Putnam's Sons, 1996
   The original Blood Type Diet book, with over two million copies sold in more than sixty-five languages.

Cook Right 4 Your Type
The Practical Kitchen Companion to Eat Right 4 Your Type
By Dr. Peter J. D'Adamo, with Catherine Whitney
G. P. Putnam's Sons, 1998 (Berkley trade paperback, 1999)

Includes over 200 original recipes, thirty-day meal plans, and guidelines for each blood type.

Live Right 4 Your Type
The Individualized Prescription for Maximizing Health, Metabolism, and Vitality in Every Stage of Your Life
By Dr. Peter J. D'Adamo, with Catherine Whitney
G. P. Putnam's Sons, 2001

A total health and lifestyle plan based on the individual variations observed for each blood type. Includes new research on the mind-body connection and the importance of blood type secretor status.

Eat Right 4 Your Type Complete Blood Type Encyclopedia
By Dr. Peter J. D'Adamo, with Catherine Whitney
Riverhead Books, 2002

The A to Z reference guide for the blood type connection to symptoms, disease, conditions, medications, vitamins, supplements, herbs, and food.

4 Your Type Pocket Guides
Blood Type, Food, Beverage and Supplement Lists
By Peter J. D'Adamo, with Catherine Whitney
Berkley Books, 2002

The Eat Right 4 Your Type Portable and Personal Blood Type Guides are pocket-sized and user-friendly. They serve as a handy reference tool while shopping, cooking, and eating out. Each book contains the food, beverage, and supplement list for each blood type plus handy tips and ideas for incorporating the Blood Type Diet into your daily life.

Eat Right 4 Your Baby
The Individualized Guide to Fertility and Maximum Health During Pregnancy, Nursing, and Your Baby's First Year
By Dr. Peter J. D'Adamo, with Catherine Whitney
G. P. Putnam's Sons, 2003

An invaluable guide for couples looking to combine the best of naturopathic and blood type science to maximize the health of mother and baby—with practical blood type–specific guidelines for achieving a healthy state before pregnancy, eating and living right during pregnancy, and how to continue in good health during baby's first year.

Dr. Peter J. D'Adamo's Eat Right 4 (for) Your Type Health Library
Arthritis: Fight It with the Blood Type Diet ®
Cancer: Fight It with the Blood Type Diet ®
Cardiovascular Disease: Fight It with the Blood Type Diet ®
Diabetes: Fight It with the Blood Type Diet ®
Fatigue: Fight It with the Blood Type Diet ®

Index

Printed in the United States
by Baker & Taylor Publisher Services